A GUTSY GIRL'S

Bible

A 21-DAY APPROACH TO HEALING THE GUT

SARAH KAY HOFFMAN

A GUTSY GIRL®
Collection

*"I've got sunshine on a cloudy day
with my girl...."*—THE TEMPTATIONS

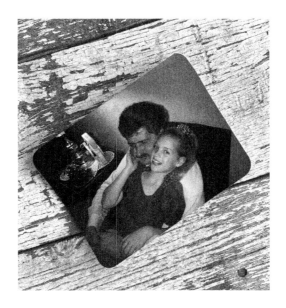

TO DAD:

Thank you for loving me as is and for never giving up your fight.
I smile when I think about your life, I thank you for pushing me
to finally finish this book, and I miss you in ways you'll never
know. Love always, Your Girl.

Contents

STAND FOR SOMETHING

I'm a country girl, through and through. I grew up on gravel roads in a small town in southern Minnesota. So even though country singer Aaron Tippin was not the one who coined this phrase, I hear his voice singing it in my head often: "You've got to stand for something or you'll fall for anything."

The challenge, of course, is in learning what you truly want to stand for. When I started my gut-healing journey, I was certain that I stood for food and lifestyle changes, and not for medications. Unfortunately, though, that didn't work, even when I desperately willed it to. At the same time, I knew that standing only for drugs and medical interventions was not for me. So in 2018, at a crossroads with my life and health, I decided to see what would happen if I put both together, combining food and lifestyle changes with medication.

And then it finally happened: I healed my gut, and I healed my life. In doing so, I realized that what I really stood for was something far greater than food, lifestyle, or medications—I stood for *empowerment*.

Today, my life is devoted to empowering women like you to make the right decisions for your body and your health. I am not a registered dietician, doctor, or professionally trained chef, but I am a Holistic Health Coach, wellness expert, gut health and healing researcher, and most importantly, a person who has lived this journey and found my own way to successful gut-healing. At the time of this writing, I am now three years in full remission from my gut-health issues; three years symptom-free.

I believe wholeheartedly that my life experiences have brought me to this place for a reason: To share my knowledge and expertise to empower *you* to make the decisions that will advance your gut-healing journey and ultimately help you to live a healthier, happier life.

Find Your Purpose

This book is titled *A Gutsy Girl's Bible,* not *The Gutsy Girl's Bible,* for a reason. What I know to be true is that there are a million ways to approach anything in life, and healing the gut is no different. My story, methods, and teachings are here to show you *a* way to go about healing, but mine is not the only way. Your journey is your own, and finding your purpose is the key to getting started on the right road.

I see you, and I know that finding purpose in this journey you're on is a struggle. You may find yourself thinking, *What's the point? Why did this happen? How did I get here?*

I want you to know you *will* find your own purpose in due time. For me personally, I know that if I had never gotten sick, I would never have learned to appreciate the art of actual good food. I would never have changed the trajectory of my career, in which I now get to do things I love on a daily basis. If I had been well, I believe getting pregnant and then staying pregnant would have been far easier—but without this journey, I would not have my angel babies, three children adopted from the foster care system. My gut-health journey has been one big learning experience. It humbled me, and it taught me to stop judging others' choices and to simply love and help in all the ways I could.

I don't have all the answers for you, but my goal with this book is to show you that *you* hold your *own* answers. I am committed to you, and I hope you are nothing less than 110% committed to yourself.

Introduction to the Gutsy Girl Approach

The gut is a delicate, intricate place, and healing the gut is extremely subjective. There are so many different gut-related diagnoses and imbalances, and just as many suggestions for how to fix them. There are hundreds of theories and ideas out there, from plant-based diets to animal-protein-only diets, from going sugar-free to focusing on "good" sugars, from FODMAP diets to detoxes to supplements, and so on. But the truth is, there is no one-size-fits-all solution. I wish there were, but I believe in bio individuality—the idea that we are all unique, that no two individuals are identical, and that not everyone will heal and thrive in the same way.

This is why *A Gutsy Girl's Bible* is *an* approach, not *the* approach, to healing the gut. In this book, I offer a basic guide to some of the gut-healing approaches I have had firsthand success with. My approach is designed to help you achieve what Dr. Steven Lamm has called the "movement from intervention to prevention."[1] The goal is to help you balance your gut over time to prevent flare-ups before they begin, so that you can spend less time managing pain and discomfort and more time enjoying life.

This book is not intended as an end-all, be-all solution or a substitute for professional medical care. It is not a long-term "diet" or a daily caloric intake plan. You won't find me laying out eating schedules or telling you how many calories to eat, because all of these things are very individualistic and depend on various factors.

This book is a guide to getting started on your own healing journey, with a focus on three main areas: diagnosis, diet, and lifestyle. The 21-day guide includes stories and inspiration from my own journey, along with prompts to help you find your own customized healing path. And if you need additional support along the way, I hope you'll join the Gutsy Girl community at facebook.com/groups/agutsygirl.

---

[1]https://pressroom.journolink.com/enzymedicauk/release/no_guts_no_glory_520

Who Is the Gutsy Girl?

Everyone is seemingly talking about "gut health" these days. But you, my friend, are no stranger to the conversation. If you're reading this book, at the very least, you have probably been struggling with some sort of gut issue that has left you feeling bloated, gassy, fatigued, irritable, sad, frustrated, and/or in some sort of physical pain. Perhaps where you find yourself today is even further along the road. You may have been suffering for a while, and perhaps a doctor has told you, "It's just IBS." Or maybe you have even received a more specific diagnosis like SIBO (small intestinal bacterial overgrowth), acid reflux, *H. pylori*, celiac disease, colitis, or diverticulitis.

Any and all of the above make you part of the Gutsy Girl club. I'm not saying it's a club you necessarily want to be part of, but chances are good that if you've nodded to any of the above, you are a part of it—at least for now. The good news is that after reading this book and taking the time to apply the strategies to your own journey, you'll be well on your way to lasting gut healing and lifelong gut health.

What's Holding You Back from Healing Your Gut?

In the beginning of gut misery, you deal with it. Why would you heal it when that would mean you'd have to let go of something? Healing your gut means you'll have to make changes, so you might not be ready. I had a similar experience a few years back, when I was unhappy with my long hair. Each time I'd go into the hairdresser's, I would say, "I'm really getting sick of my hair . . . but I can't part with it yet." Then, it would grow longer, and I would grow more frustrated. This went on for about a year, and as I threw my wet hair into a ponytail or bun each day, it got thinner and more and more tangled. Finally, my hair became so damaged that the pain point of dealing with it every day drove me to chop that rat's nest off. It was long overdue.

How overdue is healing your gut? I wanted to keep my long hair for a myriad of reasons, but in the end, I was only making my own life more difficult—just as my clients often tell me the myriad of reasons why it took them so long to realize how miserable they felt. *continued on page 14*

THE EMOTIONAL SIDE OF ILLNESS

I talk a lot about the physical side of illness, but what about the emotional side of illness? It's *rarely* talked about, but it has affected my life in ways I cannot describe, and I know it has affected your life as well. I often get emails from readers about just how lonely and stressful dealing with illness can be. One new reader recently reached out and shared, "I recently was diagnosed with UC [ulcerative colitis]. The past month has been a difficult and stressful time for me and those around me . . . My life literally has come to a screeching halt. The number of tears that I shed feeling defeated were too numerous to count. I've been struggling with feeling like it's my fault I got sick and I wasn't paying attention to my body. I've also been struggling with being now suddenly afraid of food . . . Did you ever deal with these feelings or thoughts? I want to have a healthy relationship with food and not let my illness develop into an eating disorder."

The struggle is real for those of us with chronic illness, and the emotional side of it cannot be ignored. Throughout my own experience, my emotions always ran high, and I was plagued daily by questions like "What if I *never* get better?" "Am I on the correct antibiotics?" "Should I be eating more or less?" "How did I get here?" "How can I escape?" The emotions can feel paralyzing and suffocating, and what you're feeling in your mind can take an additional toll on your body, too.

I remember on the day our son Isaiah was officially adopted—what should have been one of the happiest days of my life—my joy was clouded by deep anxiety from bloat so bad I could barely move. Don't get me wrong, it was *still* one of the happiest days of my life, but on our drive to the courthouse, I could barely breathe. I was sweating. My upper stomach was in so much pain, and hidden under my beautiful, flowing, country-girl dress, it was all bloat. I was irritable. I snapped at my husband, who is the best person in the *entire* world, for no reason. I wanted to have a serious break-down but didn't.

As I told the woman with UC who reached out recently, the emotional side of illness is oh so real.

Your tears are real. Accepting that it's a process is *very real*, but actually accepting that process is very hard to do, especially once you've been at it for months and years.

Feeling defeated is real. Your ideas that somehow it's your fault are real. Knowing that you need certain food to help you heal and avoiding others to keep you from regressing is a real thing, but the rabbit hole you'll find yourself digging into could be filled with fear toward all food.

In other words, your thoughts are all *completely* normal. Illness takes a very real toll on our emotions. In fact, I believe with all my heart that my emotional struggle was much more enduring and painful than the physical illness. Ironically, I believe the emotional side is what *kept* me from healing my physical symptoms for years.

But I also know from experience that this battle can be won by focusing on this core component: letting go of control.

CONTROL

There was a moment in time when I came to this realization through this thought: **It's not a sweet potato or rice or legumes or a cupcake or anything else that makes us (and keeps us) sick. No, instead, it's the control we try to keep around all of it and the attention we give to the details. We miss the forest for the trees.**

When I speak about control for emotional healing, I'm describ-ing the idea that no matter your circumstances, you must live life. I had been *afraid* of so many things for years. This hold was paralyzing, and living life the way I desired to live it didn't happen because of it.

I can name specific events, outings, gatherings and just about every other kind of "life moment" I have failed to participate in (whether via body or spirit) *because* of this illness.

But there is no single food, supplement or daily choice that makes or breaks healing.

The sum of the parts is always greater than the individual piece.

Understanding this and giving up that tight control will do wonders for your healing.

I've been to every imaginable doctor and nutritionist, and I've learned that you will *never* find the help you need to heal emotionally there (unless you need medication, of course).

You might find it via therapy, but how do you *really* find it? You must dig deep, in dark places, and uncover the root to all emotional ties. It is in these places where, once you peel back the layers, your health will greatly improve.

These dark places are, in fact, the sum of the parts of all your experiences (from birth to now). It wasn't until I sought out my past and explored my life's experiences that I was able to heal and move forward in the present.

Each time I was "stuck" on something or someone, I spent time in my journal and therapy peeling back the words, thoughts, and actions associated with it in order to help myself move forward.

This is what I'm talking about with true, ultimate, and everlasting healing.

Emotions that stay stuffed will keep your health issue(s) stuck.

But in the meantime, know that there is nothing wrong with the way you're feeling, and be real good to yourself today. You deserve it.

Dig deep and ask yourself, what's holding you back from healing your gut? It's always something, and the longer you don't address that something, the bigger of a problem it will become. Excuses are always convenient when you're afraid to take grand steps forward, but like the ends of my long hair, excuses remain dead. I never magically came to love my long hair, and your gut won't just magically heal.

Rid yourself of your excuses, dig deep today, and ask:

What's holding me back from healing my gut?

A 21-Day Journey

They say it takes 21 days to create a habit, and I've found that 21 days is the perfect length for starting on a new lifestyle plan like this one. If you can stay consistent for 21 days and find that what you're doing *works*, you'll feel motivated to do another 21 days. And if you need to pivot and go in a new direction, 21 days is short enough that you can easily reevaluate, readjust, and start fresh.

During this 21-day journey, you will take small steps each day, such as experimenting with dietary changes, making sure to drink at least 8 cups of water and get enough sleep, adding daily exercise into your routine, and working with your doctor, nutritionist, or other medical provider to find the right supplements, medications, or lifestyle changes for you.

Journaling is also an important part of the process, so this book includes plenty of space for jotting down your thoughts. You can use this space to keep track of your progress, record notes on your menstrual cycle, and write thoughts of gratitude and/or healing mantras.

The 21-day journey is designed to help you start off on the right track with a few key goals in mind. First, it's essential to get yourself an accurate diagnosis. "Dr. Google" will not suffice, nor will a misdiagnosis from a doctor. Without the critical first step of an accurate diagnosis, you'll be spinning your wheels forever. I did. For more on getting the diagnostic information you need, see page 21.

Once you have an accurate diagnosis, you can begin the initial repair of your gut. Repairing damage to your gut may require a short-term dose of antibiotics, a longer-term course of medication, some type of probiotic, or other supplements and herbs, depending on your individual condition and needs. After the accurate diagnosis and initial repair, you must rebuild your gut health.

But getting an accurate diagnosis, repairing, and rebuilding your health are just the beginning, and they could even be called the "easy" parts. Once you've made the decision to start, all you have to do is follow the protocols you've set. The harder part—and the ultimate goal of this journey—is to *thrive*. What is the point of living merely to survive? We should never accept a life where we are just "getting by." The goal is to thrive, and this starts with our greatest treasure: our health.

I've found that in order to thrive, it's critical to focus on five main areas, which are easy to remember using the acronym **P.R.E.S.S.**:

1. **PURPOSE:** Find yours. Live it.
2. **RELATIONSHIPS:** Work on them, remove the ones that don't work, and fight for the rest.
3. **EXERCISE:** Not too much, not too little. This one was huge for me.
4. **STRESS MANAGEMENT:** The gut-brain connection is massive. Until you learn to truly control stress, you will never thrive.
5. **SLEEP:** I've always hated the saying, "You can sleep when you die." A lack of sleep has a trickle effect, and its negative consequences for me included chronic illness. Make sleep a priority or you'll suffer your own consequences.

Begin this journey by committing 21 days, and then make a plan to P.R.E.S.S. on and continue along the healing path. But please don't mistake this plan as a fast track to overnight results. Real, long-term healing takes time,

HOW TO USE THIS GUIDE

I recommend that you read this entire book before beginning your 21-day journey or putting anything into practice. The reason is simple: There is a ton of information here, and before you begin to take action, you will need to be mentally and physically prepared.

Mentally, you need to be ready, willing, and able to make a change. These 21 days are *not* for the faint of heart, but I can guarantee you will, at the very least, begin to get some answers. You also need to ensure you can devote this time for *you*. For women, this can be a tough task—we are leaders, goers, doers, and makers. But to get the most out of your healing journey, please stop and take some time for yourself and your gut. If at all possible, do *not* overbook yourself during the 21 days. These 21 days are a time for you to figure it all out so you can begin moving on with your life. Not only will you be exploring your relationship with food, you will also dabble into your thoughts, engage in movement, address your stress levels, and learn as much as you can about lifestyle and diet.

Physically, you need to ensure you have the appropriate foods and resources. About a week before you begin, stock your fridge, freezer, and pantry with the items you'll need. It's also a good idea to begin weaning yourself off the things you are most dependent on about a week in advance. If you are highly addicted to sugar, for example, you will want to start reducing it little by little. Don't binge just because you know a 21-day commitment is coming.

Once you are ready, simply begin on Day 1. Remember, everything starts at the beginning.

but you should not feel discouraged by that, because you now have all the pieces you need to start, one step at a time. Each day is progress. I am living proof.

DISCLAIMER: *I am not a professional chef. I am not a registered dietitian or doctor. I am a Holistic Health Coach, wellness expert, and lover of food as a way to heal the gut while soaking up all the beauty that life truly gives. My intentions are not to substitute for the advice given by a licensed healthcare professional. You are ultimately responsible for any and all actions taken. Please review the disclaimer on the copyright page prior to starting.*

A Gutsy Girl's 21-Day Healing Method

Healing my gut was a long journey, with many false starts along the way. There is so much information available in books and on the Internet about how to heal the gut and how to heal chronic illnesses, but unfortunately, much of it is conflicting information, and sometimes it feels like you need a medical degree to understand it! The biggest issue, though, is that none of the information was written *for you*. It's all for a generalized population, and you are not general; you are one of a kind.

When I finally found success, it all boiled down to two main ideas:

Simplify and **Customize**.

When it came to healing my gut and then staying well for years afterward, **simplifying** things was key. It's like digestion: The reason we chew our food 30 to 40 times prior to swallowing is that it breaks down our food into the simplest form possible, making it easier to digest. The more we break down the principles of gut healing into a simple, linear format, the easier it is to implement the ideas and heal faster.

That's why this book distills my advice and experience down into a step-by-step, 21-day plan. It's also why you'll find what I like to call "Creations," rather than standardized recipes, at the end of this book. I am not Martha Stewart—I'm not even a professional blogger who creates big, beautiful recipes for gut-healing meal plans. Part of what helped me heal was *cutting out* those complicated recipes and replacing them with simple concoctions that could be easily customized to fit my mood or use the ingredients I already had on hand. While a recipe with 12 ingredients, 7 of which are "good for the gut," might be a lovely dinner, when you're beginning on your healing journey, it can also be overwhelming and will likely make you more confused than ever. If there's one thing I hope you'll take away from this book, it's that mastering the art of simplifying will help you to make huge progress toward healing.

The second key idea here is **customization**. Never, ever, in the history of gut healing has there been one *right way* for healing. There is no universal set of supplements, medications, or dietary guidelines that will work for everyone, or even work for one person at all times. How many times have you picked up a book and crossed your fingers in hopes that the information you were about to read was *the* information you had been desperately waiting for? Inevitably, though, you find yourself back at square one, but with the added frustration of feeling like you've lost time or even reversed your progress. This is because there is no book on the market that was customized uniquely for you—not even this one.

I'm not interested in making you feel like there is one correct way toward healing. Instead, in this book, I want to empower you to always and forever customize everything *for you*. In the pages that follow, I'll give you the tools to do this. Throughout your 21-day journey, you'll be choosing the tactics that work best for you on any given day, and journaling along the way to help you reflect on your own unique needs.

If you can remember these two words, "simplify" and "customize," as you read this book and beyond, what you're going to be able to do will amaze you!

Why 21 Days?

You may be wondering, why is this plan 21 days long? Why not just make it a month, or even shorten it to a week? But the 21-day length was set very intentionally. The idea was born in January 2007, when I did my first true detox. The program was 21 days long, and as I neared the end of it, I felt the best I ever had. Like magic, I felt 100% around Day 19. But when I went back to my old ways on Day 22, misery set in immediately. This was when I first realized that in just 21 days, one could learn a lot about their body and symptoms.

If you've been feeling miserable for a while, you will likely start seeing at least one positive change around the one-week mark. However, a week is not enough time to practice your new habits, track them, and journal their effects. But on the flip side, a month seems to be too long for most people to stick with a new plan. We tend to commit to things more easily if the commitment is for a shorter time. I've found that 21 days is the perfect length of time to both encourage commitment and see real results.

EVERY DAY, FOR 21 DAYS

This part is *very* important, so pay attention! There is a secret to these 21 days and to the success of your journey: When you cut corners and "cheat," the *only* person you are cheating is yourself.

If I say it's important that you do x, y, and z on a daily basis, but you choose not to, that's your prerogative. However, at the end of 21 days, you may find that things haven't turned out the way you had hoped or intended, and you must be willing to take full accountability for that.

When I finally healed myself once and for all, it was because I had learned the value and power of answering to *myself*. It's not easy to hear, but the reality is that when you are silently suffering with gas, bloat, and diarrhea, *no one cares as much as you do*. In fact, others may not even believe you or give you the time of day for complaining. You will have no one to answer to on this 21-day journey but yourself. If you want to heal, uncover answers, and live a healthier and happier life, you'll need to start by accepting 21 days of self-discipline.

Each day of your journey will include a list of daily actions that are critical to take, optional actions to consider, easily customizable food "Creations" to try, and a Real Thought for the day. Along the way, I'll also share snippets from my own personal journey to encourage you on yours. The 21-day plan takes a holistic approach to gut healing by focusing on three key areas at once: Diagnosis, Diet, and Lifestyle. These are what I like to call the Three Pillars of Ultimate Gut Healing.

Three Pillars of Ultimate Gut Healing

After years of struggling to understand my own gut-health issues, I eventually learned that the three pillars of any healing journey are diagnosis, diet, and lifestyle. You'll never heal your gut by focusing on any one of these alone in a silo; you need to address all three together in order to find your way forward.

I first came up with the idea of three pillars after completing school at the Institute for Integrative Nutrition, where I learned all about diet and lifestyle as a means for healing and living more vibrantly. What I learned there was a huge help in understanding my own gut issues, but there was a third key factor that also made a big difference: receiving a SIBO diagnosis after years of misery. This was an essential piece I needed to solve the puzzle and get my health on the right track.

My three pillars combine Western and alternative thinking, and each school of thought is applied where I feel it does the best job. For example, Western medicine is great for diagnosis, but you're not likely to get very far with your family doctor or even your gastroenterologist on the lifestyle side of things, because they have neither the time nor the specialized knowledge to help you with that pillar. No part of the equation is easy, but you'll need all three pillars working together to support you on your 21-day journey.

DIAGNOSIS

No matter where you are or how you got sick, you must know that things can change. But first, if you are self-diagnosing, you must stop. Too many people use "Dr. Google" to diagnose themselves. I don't blame you for this—with all the information available on the Internet, it's easy to think, "A doctor's diagnosis could take a long time and a lot of money, I'll just change XYZ and see how I respond." But oftentimes, all this does is prolong the process and keep you from ultimate healing.

It's also important to note that not just any educated guess will do—to find the right path to healing, you need the *right* diagnosis. As I was getting ready to be discharged from the ER once, I asked the doctor, "So, what did you find to be the cause?" He replied, "We don't know." However, he said, "We think it's one of a couple things, so we ordered prescriptions for both, just in case."

When I reviewed the paperwork and what they diagnosed me with, I laughed. They just guessed. I never went to pick up the prescriptions. Educated guesses do not suffice, and popping pills and following "medical plans" without accurate information can be more damaging than helpful.

I know because I've lived it.

Every single day, I am asked, "How do I know if I have SIBO, adrenal fatigue, colitis, celiac, and so on?" *continued on page 24*

A Gutsy Girl's Three Pillars of Ultimate Gut Healing

My three pillars of ultimate gut healing are unique in the sense that they combine Western and alternative viewpoints.

THREE PILLARS OF ULTIMATE GUT HEALING		
		LIFESTYLE (most difficult pillar to conquer; can include everything from movement to stress management, therapy to personal care items with or without supplements and/or medications)
DIAGNOSIS (not Dr. Google)	**DIET** (the right diet for your body)	

There was a time when I spoke loud and clear:
Diet and lifestyle versus drugs and medications.

And you know what? I wish that could be the case for everyone. I truly do. In fact, I tried to make it my own scenario for years. Doing so was detrimental. Why? Because it only added years to my healing journey.

Yes, years.

The reason is that I failed on two very important levels:
- Diagnosis.
- Understanding that drugs and medications could be part of the lifestyle equation.

But I couldn't see this clearly until after I put in one of my final puzzle pieces; the SIBO diagnosis.

No, it wasn't the final piece, but it was a huge piece I needed in the end.
This journal can help you uncover your own missing puzzle pieces.

Scan this QR code with your smartphone camera for more information for your journey.

DIAGNOSIS *(NOT DR. GOOGLE)*

The **diagnosis pillar** alone can take months (and even years, which was the case for me).

One of the most common series of questions I am asked includes:
What tests should I ask for? And what is doing a test for XYZ like? Should I get another opinion? Do you think this is really what's going on with me? What do my test results/numbers mean? Could there be more? Etc.

Regardless of the questions you're asking, you must ask them and get the appropriate tests instead of relying on Dr. Google. Never rely on the Internet. Your gut-healing efforts will be expedited once you know for sure.

DIET

The **diet pillar** is about figuring out what works for you.

Lean in closely when I tell you this secret. Are you ready? Dialing in the diet is a test of will, determination, and patience. Why? Because it will (and must!) be 100% customized for you.

Everyone wants to be gluten-free or dairy-free, keto, paleo, or vegetarian. Diet molds never work, and the reason is that we are all different.

Figuring out what will work for you, though, is critical in overall gut healing because 70%+ of your immune system lies in your gut. Your overall well-being is related to how healthy your gut is: that is, digestion and gut bacteria.

LIFESTYLE

The **lifestyle pillar** includes things like movement (exercise, workouts), stress reduction, increased sleep, spirituality, relationships, safer skincare, makeup, and body care, nontoxic home living, and all other critical lifestyle factors that may or may not include supplements and/or medications.

This is the part of the equation everyone knows needs work, but no one wants to admit.

Once someone has an appropriate diagnosis and then figures out the diet that's right for them, many times symptoms still exist.

The lifestyle piece is the why. It is by far the most difficult pillar to conquer.

The simple answer is, "You are diagnosed with it." If you are struggling with painful symptoms and want to begin healing, **go get tested, immediately.** Don't wait any longer. Stop consulting with Dr. Google. Your condition likely shares symptoms with a thousand others, and the longer you dwell on them without knowing a true diagnosis, the more damage you are doing.

It's also important to know that **you're *not* insane, and you don't have to let anyone make you feel that way.** All too often friends, family members, and even doctors can make you feel like your symptoms are not real or are your own fault. I felt insane a lot because, even after my diagnoses, people would tell me it was all in my head when I knew "healthy" things like avocado, apples, garlic, and onion made feel horrible. But guess what? I wasn't insane. Today, I'm eating all those foods with zero problems, because I finally got the right diagnosis to allow me to heal my gut. The definition of insanity is doing the same things over and over and expecting a different result, so you're only insane if you continue to self-diagnose when you are getting no results.

The diagnosis piece can take months (or even years, which was the case for me), but it's an essential first step in your healing process. If you're scared, I understand. Start by getting yourself a gut-healing journal so you can stay organized, and then read on for more on the types of digestive health testing you may want to explore.

What's Wrong with Me?

Some of the most common questions I am asked include:

What tests should I ask for? And what is doing a test for XYZ like? Should I get another opinion? Do you think this is really what's going on with me? What do my test results/numbers mean? Could there be more? Of course, every situation is unique, so to answer these questions accurately, you must speak with a qualified health provider and get the appropriate tests. Your gut-healing efforts will be expedited once you know for sure. There are a huge number of different disorders that can affect the digestive system, and many share similar symptoms.

Here are some of the most common issues you may need to be tested for or may be diagnosed with:

DIAGNOSIS	WHAT IT MEANS
Barrett's esophagus	Barrett's esophagus is often diagnosed in people who have long-term gastroesophageal reflux disease (GERD). Only a small percentage of people with GERD will develop Barrett's esophagus, but it's important because it is associated with an increased risk of developing esophageal cancer.
Candida	Candida is a fungus, which is a form of yeast, a very small amount of which lives in your mouth and intestines. Its job is to aid with digestion and nutrient absorption. An overproduction of candida breaks down the wall of the intestine and penetrates the bloodstream, releasing toxic by-products into your body and causing leaky gut. This can lead to many different health problems ranging from digestive issues to depression.
Celiac disease	Celiac disease is a serious autoimmune disorder that can occur in genetically predisposed people where the ingestion of gluten leads to damage in the small intestine. About 1 in 100 people worldwide (estimated) are affected by celiac disease. The *only* treatment currently for celiac disease is adherence to a strict gluten-free diet.[2]
Clostridioides[3] *difficile* (*C. diff.*)	Many know this by the term *C. diff. Clostridioides difficile* is a Gram-positive, spore-forming bacterium. It is an opportunistic pathogen, infecting the colon of patients following antibiotic treatment. *C. difficile* produces two toxins, TcdA and TcdB, which damage intestinal cells and cause inflammation in the gut.
Constipation	I included this one, even though I believe that chronic constipation almost always goes hand in hand with something else on this list. Chronic constipation is infrequent bowel movements or difficult passage of stools that persists for several weeks or longer. Constipation typically occurs with fewer than three bowel movements a week. Constipation would be a 1 to 3 on the Bristol Stool Chart.

[2] https://celiac.org/about-the-foundation/featured-news/2016/08/20-things-you-might-not-know-about-celiac-disease/#:~:text=1%20in%20100%20people%20worldwide,of%20developing%20celiac%20disease%20themselves
[3] http://www.thelancet.com/journals/laninf/article/PIIS1473-3099(19)30177-X/fulltext

Crohn's disease	There are different types of Crohn's disease that affect different areas of the GI tract. The most common form of Crohn's, ileocolitis affects the end of the small intestine (the ileum) and the large intestine (the colon). Symptoms include diarrhea and cramping or pain in the right lower part or middle of the abdomen. This type is often accompanied by significant weight loss.
Diarrhea	The opposite of constipation is diarrhea. In most cases, diarrhea lasts a couple of days. But when diarrhea lasts for weeks, it can indicate a serious disorder, such as a persistent infection, inflammatory bowel disease, or a less serious condition, such as irritable bowel syndrome. Going back to the Bristol Stool Chart, diarrhea would be in the range of a 5 to 7 (mostly a "7").
Diverticulitis	Diverticula are small, bulging pouches that can form in the lining of your digestive system. You'll find them most often in the lower part of the large intestine (colon). When one or more of the pouches become inflamed or infected, it is known as diverticulitis, which can cause severe stomach bulging, pain, fever, nausea, and a marked change in your bowel habits.
Escherichia coli (*E. coli*)	*Escherichia coli* (*E. coli*) bacteria normally live in the intestines of healthy people and animals. Most varieties of *E. coli* are harmless or cause relatively brief diarrhea. But a few particularly nasty strains, such as *E. coli* O157:H7, can cause severe abdominal cramps, bloody diarrhea, and vomiting.
Gallstones	Gallstones are stones or lumps that develop in the gallbladder or bile duct when certain substances harden. There are approximately 20 million Americans with gallstones.[4]
Gastroenteritis (stomach flu)	Gastroenteritis is an inflammation of the gastrointestinal tract (the pathway responsible for digestion that includes the mouth, esophagus, stomach, and intestines). You may have heard "stomach flu," even though it may not be related to influenza.

---

[4]https://www.worldgastroenterology.org/publications/e-wgn/e-wgn-expert-point-of-view-articles-collection/the-growing-global-burden-of-gallstone-disease

Gastroesophageal reflux (GER) + **Gastroesophageal reflux disease** (GERD)	Gastroesophageal reflux (GER) happens when your stomach contents come back up into your esophagus, causing heartburn (also called acid reflux). GERD is a long-lasting and more serious form of GER.
Gluten sensitivity	Your blood test for celiac disease came back negative, but you still don't feel well. Now what? If you have been suffering from symptoms that seem related to gluten, it may be possible that you have non-celiac gluten sensitivity ("gluten sensitivity"). Research estimates that 18 million Americans have gluten sensitivity. That's six times the amount of Americans who have celiac disease.[5]
Helicobacter pylori (*H. pylori*)	*Helicobacter pylori* (aka *H. pylori*) is a bacteria that has been around for at least 200,000 years. If you have this infection, you're actually most likely not to have any symptoms. But having this bacteria living in your body can make your risk of developing gastric cancer up to six times higher. Plus, *H. pylori* bacteria is often at the root of other major digestive problems, like peptic ulcers and gastritis. So not only can *H. pylori* cause stomach ulcers, it can also cause ulcers in your esophagus or small intestine.
Hemorrhoids	Hemorrhoids are usually caused by increased pressure due to pregnancy, being overweight, or straining during bowel movements. By midlife, hemorrhoids often become an ongoing complaint. By age 50, about half the population has experienced one or more of the classic symptoms, which include rectal pain, itching, bleeding, and possibly prolapse (hemorrhoids that protrude through the anal canal). Although hemorrhoids are rarely dangerous, they can be a recurrent and painful intrusion.[6]

---

[5]https://www.rn.com/headlines-in-health/gluten-its-not-for-everyone/#:~:text=It%20is%20estimated%20that%2018,diagnosed%20with%20a%20gluten%20allergy.
[6]https://www.health.harvard.edu/diseases-and-conditions/hemorrhoids_and_what_to_do_about_them

Inflammatory bowel disease (IBD)	IBD stands for "inflammatory bowel disease." It is classified as a disease, not a syndrome. Unlike IBS, IBD causes changes in bowel tissue and increases your chances for colorectal cancer. IBD involves chronic inflammation on all or part of the digestive tract, and it primarily includes ulcerative colitis and Crohn's disease. There is currently no *cure* for IBD. However, the disease can go into remission.
Irritable bowel syndrome (IBS)	Irritable bowel syndrome (IBS) is known as "spastic colon." Since it is a syndrome, it is a set or range of symptoms that may fall into the defining category, Irritable bowel syndrome. IBS, unlike inflammatory bowel disease (IBD), does *not* cause tissue inflammation. In other words, if you were to be "scoped," doctors would *not* find tissue inflammation, scarring, etc. from IBS alone.
Lactose intolerance	Lactose intolerance can cause various symptoms, including bloating, diarrhea, and abdominal cramps. It is the body's inability to digest lactose, the main carbohydrate in dairy products. People with lactose intolerance don't make enough of the enzyme lactase, which is needed to digest lactose. Dairy is one tricky devil, though. Be sure to review my list of 100 dairy sources and alternate names.
Leaky gut syndrome	In the simplest terms, leaky gut syndrome is when the cells that make up the lining of the intestinal tract become so inflamed that the gut lining becomes more permeable than it's meant to be. This, in turn, causes things that shouldn't get through to the bloodstream to seep through, resulting in a myriad of health problems.
Pancreatitis	Pancreatitis is inflammation of the pancreas. Acute pancreatitis is short term and may go away in a few days with treatment. Chronic, or long-lasting, pancreatitis can get worse over time and cause lasting damage.
Parasites	This is not an appetizing picture to paint, but it affects people worldwide, so it should not be overlooked. A parasite is an organism that lives on or in a host organism and gets its food from or at the expense of its host. There are three main classes of parasites that can cause disease in humans: protozoa, helminths, and ectoparasites.

Small intestinal bacterial overgrowth (SIBO)	SIBO stands for "small intestinal bacterial overgrowth." Those with SIBO have an abnormally large amount of bacteria in the small intestine. This bacteria is not inherently good or bad; it's just not where it should be in the correct amounts.
Stomach ulcers	Stomach ulcers (gastric ulcers) are open sores that develop on the lining of the stomach. Ulcers can also occur in part of the intestine just beyond the stomach. They are duodenal ulcers. Stomach and duodenal ulcers are sometimes called peptic ulcers.
Ulcerative colitis	Ulcerative colitis is an inflammatory bowel disease (IBD) that causes long-lasting inflammation and ulcers (sores) in your digestive tract. It affects the innermost lining of your large intestine (colon) and rectum. Symptoms usually develop over time, rather than suddenly. Doctors often classify ulcerative colitis according to its location, and the classifications include ulcerative proctitis (which is what I was diagnosed with in 2008), proctosigmoiditis, left-sided colitis, pancolitis, and acute severe ulcerative colitis.

What Can I Expect at the Doctor?

Unless you take control of the situation and go to your doctor's appointment *ultra-prepared*, you are not likely to get the outcome you're looking for. This is the cold, hard truth. If you have high expectations heading into the appointment but haven't done your prep work, you'll be left with even more frustration and confusion than when you entered the clinic doors.

In order to have your high expectations met (and you should!), be prepared and bring the doctor your full medical history, any notes you've taken on the timing and severity of your symptoms, and an idea about what specific tests you are requesting from your doctor so that they can help you in the best ways possible.

If you are prepared for the appointment, here are some tests your doctor might order to have performed:

Blood Draw and/or Skin Prick Test	These tests are looking for *true* allergies.
Celiac Blood Test	A blood test that looks for higher than normal levels of certain antibodies in the blood. Diagnostic for celiac disease.
Colonoscopy	During a colonoscopy, a long, thin, flexible tool (endoscope) is inserted via the rectum in order to view the bowels and colon.
Complete Blood Count (CBC)	A general blood test for overall markers.
DUTCH Complete Hormone Panel	Extremely comprehensive hormone test to tell you everything about the current state of your hormone levels.
Endoscopy	During an endoscopy, a long, thin, flexible tool (endoscope) is inserted via the mouth. There is a light, video camera, and telescope on the tool and, when inserted, it travels down your internal organs. This allows the doctor to look closely at your upper digestive system.
Functional Adrenal Stress Profile	Saliva test that measures cortisol levels at various times throughout the day.
GI Map	Comprehensive stool sample that measures a variety of bacteria (including *H. pylori*), parasites, viruses, fungi/yeast, antibiotic resistance genes, and several intestinal health markers.
OAT (Great Plains Lab Organic Acids Test)	Provides an accurate evaluation of intestinal yeast and bacteria. It also includes markers for vitamin and mineral levels, oxidative stress, and neurotransmitter levels, and it is the only OAT to include markers for oxalates, which are highly correlated with many chronic illnesses.[7]
Small Intestinal Bacterial Overgrowth (SIBO) Test	Breath testing that can determine the levels of hydrogen and/or methane in your intestines.
Thyroid Panel	Blood test to determine thyroid levels. Note: When you get this testing done, be sure to ask for more than just your TSH levels. Ask for "the full thyroid panel."

---

[7] https://goldenhealthholistics.com/great-plains-lab-organic-acids-test-oat

COLONOSCOPY AND ENDOSCOPY

People ask me all the time about colonoscopy and endoscopy. I say, when in doubt, just do it. When a client comes to work with me because their gut is a complete mess, I always recommend a trip to a gastroenterologist to find out if they should in fact be "scoped." The reason? The more we know, the better. Knowledge is power.

A colonoscopy and/or endoscopy can help your doctor to identify whether your problem lies in the upper or lower digestive tract. During an endoscopy, a long, thin, flexible tool called an endoscope is inserted via the mouth. There is a light, video camera, and telescope on the tool, and it travels down through your digestive organs to give an internal view. A colonoscopy uses that same tool, but it is inserted via the rectum in order to view the bowels and colon.

If something like colitis is suspected, your doctor will suggest a colonoscopy. If celiac disease or another upper-digestive-tract disorder is suspected, you'll have an endoscopy. Depending on your symptoms, your doctor may also recommend both. These tests are the best way to identify a whole host of specific gut issues, including celiac disease, Crohn's disease, colitis, polyps, general inflammation, ulcers, abnormal growths, and more.

If you've been suffering from digestive issues, the best time to get a colonoscopy or endoscopy is now, even if you're not in the midst of an active flare-up. Unless it's an emergency test, you'll rarely end up timing a colonoscopy or endoscopy to coincide with a flare-up, but that doesn't mean the test will be any less effective.

HOW DO I PREPARE FOR A COLONOSCOPY OR ENDOSCOPY?

If you're only having an endoscopy, there's not much you'll need to worry about in terms of preparation. Just adhere to your doctor's instructions about fasting before the procedure and about any medications or over-the-counter drugs you may be using.

The preparation for a colonoscopy is more involved. It's not fun, nor glamorous, but it's important that you follow the doctor's instructions. Your doctor may advise you to stick to a special diet for a few days before the test, including avoiding nuts, seeds, fiber, grains, and blue, red, and purple foods. You'll be given a "prep liquid," a laxative that will help to completely empty your bowels. The process is unpleasant, but you can't cheat here—it all needs to come out. The procedure is very quick. You'll be given IV fluids and then anesthesia. The actual scoping process takes around 20 minutes, and you'll likely need to stay in recovery for about an hour. If you had an endoscopy, you might burp a little or feel a slightly sore throat. If you had a colonoscopy, be prepared to be a tootin' house! It's okay, the air is just coming out. You'll need to have someone available to pick you up and bring you home, since you'll be a little out of it for the rest of the day from the anesthesia. After the procedure, do everything you can to ensure your bowels will bounce back to normal as soon as possible. For me, this included drinking lots of water, taking my probiotic, and eating a lot of food containing fiber, accompanied by enzymes and HCL.

WHAT WILL I FIND OUT AND WHEN WILL I BE TOLD?

When you wake up, you'll probably get a general report on what the doctor saw, for example, if the scope identified something that needed to be removed immediately or biopsied, they might have opted to do that while you were already under anesthesia. If they needed to take any samples, you'll have to wait for the follow-up reports from your doctor. Once you've had your follow-up, if anything feels off, don't hesitate to get a second opinion on either the procedure itself or the results.

These procedures can feel invasive, but do not let anyone scare you into *not* getting these tests done. They can save your life or, at least, help guide you toward the answers you may have been searching for for years.

I advise you to get all necessary blood and other medical tests out of the way before changing your diet to heal your gut.

Why? Some blood tests (like the one that tests for celiac) rely on the fact that you are consuming gluten on a regular basis. Other tests like endoscopies and colonoscopies also are more accurate in identifying the underlying issues when you're consuming a nonrestricted diet.

Be Your Own Advocate

It seems obvious, but in the search for a real diagnosis, you must be your own advocate. You know your own body better than anyone, and you will know when the answers you're getting don't seem right. I get messages from people with IBS and IBD who are tired, frustrated, and completely over the runaround their practitioner is giving them, and I've been there, too.

For example, I recently heard from a woman who was suffering from painful stomach issues and bloating. A doctor had diagnosed her with IBS about 20 years ago after testing produced inconclusive results. Her current doctor had not ordered any further testing and wasn't able to give her helpful dietary guidance, but was prescribing antidepressants, which she did not feel comfortable taking.

It sounds like some sort of joke, but sadly, it is not, and cases like this are all too common. In order to get real answers and come up with a sensible healing plan, she would need to find a doctor willing to listen to her concerns and work with her, including doing more testing, if necessary, rather than discounting her pain and searching for a "quick fix." The only way to get out of your own personal hell is to be your own advocate. There are doctors and providers (both Western and alternative) who *will* help you, but you must find one who is willing to listen and speak up for what you need.

If you find yourself today in a similar place to the reader who reached out to me, don't give up. Do not lose hope. Advocate for yourself and keep searching for the right, real, and accurate diagnosis. It's there to find.

IBS VS. IBD: WHAT'S THE DIFFERENCE?

I am asked all the time what the difference is between IBS and IBD. While people tend to use the terms interchangeably and they share many of the same symptoms, there are major differences between the two.

WHAT IS IBS?

IBS stands for "irritable bowel syndrome." Most people with IBS will never develop IBD, but most people with IBD have IBS symptoms. IBS is known as "spastic colon," and it's a "syndrome," which means it isn't categorized as a disease; rather, it's a set of symptoms that all fall into the category of irritable bowel syndrome. IBS, unlike IBD, does not cause tissue inflammation, so if you were to be scoped, doctors would not find tissue inflammation or scarring from IBS alone.

Even though there is no permanent damage done with IBS, it still can cause day-to-day pain, discomfort, and misery for those who battle it. "According to the International Foundation for Functional Gastrointestinal Disorders, IBS affects at least 10% to 20% of adults in the U.S.—mostly women—and is second only to the common cold as a cause of absenteeism from work."[1] (And now you know why I'm so passionate about helping women in particular!)

Finally, IBS usually begins in late adolescence or early adult life, and most often at times of emotional stress.

WHAT ARE THE SYMPTOMS OF IBS?

When it comes to IBS symptoms, everyone is different. Some have the IBS-C (constipation) version, others have the IBS-D (diarrhea) version, and still others have the alternating version, which includes both constipation and diarrhea. But in general, IBS symptoms may include:

- abdominal pain

[1] https://www.townsendletter.com/FebMarch2014/IBS0214.html

- constipation
- diarrhea
- both constipation and diarrhea, alternating
- gas
- bloat
- mucus in stool

WHAT IS IBD?

IBD stands for "inflammatory bowel disease." Unlike IBS, IBD causes changes in bowel tissue and increases your chances for colorectal cancer.[2] IBD involves chronic inflammation on all or part of the digestive tract, and it primarily includes ulcerative colitis and Crohn's disease. IBD affects about 1.6 million Americans, with about 70,000 new patients being diagnosed each year.[3]

WHAT ARE THE SYMPTOMS OF IBD?

- severe diarrhea
- pain
- fatigue
- weight loss
- bleeding and/or black stools
- vomiting
- anemia
- fevers

HOW DO I KNOW IF I HAVE IBS OR IBD?

First things first: stop Googling. If you're not sure whether you have IBS or IBD, start by finding a great doctor. If you can, seek out a naturopathic/

_____

[2]https://www.mayoclinic.org/diseases-conditions/irritable-bowel-syndrome/symptoms-causes/syc-20360016
[3]https://www.crohnscolitisfoundation.org/campus-connection/what-is-ibd

holistic doctor (MD). If you choose a traditional Western medicine doctor, seek out referrals first. Trust me, I spent far too long trying to find a good one.

Based on a physical, your symptoms, and more, your doctor will determine if you need a colonoscopy and/or endoscopy or other further testing, including blood samples, stool samples, and X-rays. These diagnostic tests will help your doctor to reach a final conclusion.

TREATMENTS FOR IBS VS. IBD

If your doctor determines that you do have IBS or IBD, your treatment options may include a combination of dietary changes, stress management, acupucture, antidepressant medication, and pain relievers. For IBD, your doctor may also want to prescribe steroids or other medications like low-dose naltrexone, Remicade, Humira, aminosalicylates, or metronidazole (Flagyl). Surgery may also be an option. For IBS sufferers, antidiarrheal medications can also help.

It's also important to remember that there are two types of IBS and IBD: IBS/IBD-D comes with diarrhea, while IBS/IBD-C causes constipation. You may have one or the other, or a form that toggles between the two. When making dietary changes to help address your IBS or IBD, keep in mind that diarrhea and constipation each require a different approach.

For Diarrhea:

- Avoid nuts until diarrhea has cleared.
- Be very cautious with raw nuts, fruits, vegetables, etc.
- Try high-protein dairy like homemade kefir and yogurt to help bulk the stool (*not* high-fat dairy, which can aggravate diarrhea). (Note: You must make your own; kefir and yogurt from the grocery store will not have the same effect.)
- Avoid Epsom salt baths.

- Limit vitamin C powder.
- Avoid extra magnesium.

For Constipation:

- Ensure you are eating enough gelatinous, high-protein meats and fats, such as liver, and less muscle meats, like boneless, skinless chicken breast. Avoid high-protein dairy, which can aggravate constipation.
- Drink lots of juice made from high-magnesium fruit and vegetables, such as oranges, celery, apples, carrots, cabbage, beets, and greens.
- Try a magnesium supplement.

While the specific foods may vary from one type of IBS/IBD to the other, fundamentally you can heal both in the same way: by focusing on both diet *and* lifestyle. If you are following this 21-day plan carefully and eating top-quality, unprocessed foods, most of your diarrhea and constipation will naturally improve.

Once I Have My Diagnosis, What's Next?

Once you have your diagnosis, it's time to get to work. I don't say this to scare you, but I promise you'll never fully heal if you don't put the time, energy, and effort into it.

Think of it like this: Your computer breaks down, so you take it to the technician to get fixed. When the computer has been fixed, the technician tells you that for the computer to remain in good standing, you'll need to be sure to back it up each night, complete the prompted updates, and run a thorough scan on it each month to be sure no viruses have crept in again. You want your computer to stay healthy and well, so you listen to the technician, even though it does require a little bit of work.

Healing your gut is no different—and your health is so much more valuable than the computer you wouldn't think twice about giving some extra TLC.

After your diagnosis, listen to what the doctor told you and begin taking any recommended medications and supplements. Will they always be the right ones at the right dose? No. But if a doctor has prescribed them, then start there, and work with your provider to make any needed adjustments along the way.

You'll also need to focus on dietary changes—this is the second pillar of healing your gut. Finally, you'll want to zero-in on your lifestyle. Go all in on this one.

Your diagnosis is only the beginning.

DIET

Once you've gotten on the right track with a correct diagnosis, the second pillar is figuring out the best diet for your body. Don't listen to the doctor who tells you food does not matter. You don't have to be a doctor, nutritionist, or scientist to know and understand that food does matter. In fact, with a little trial and error in the beginning of your journey, you'll quickly witness how much it matters firsthand.

And don't listen to anyone—not your mom, dad, sister, aunt, or best friend's third cousin—who tells you that any templated diet on Earth is right for you. Dialing in to the diet that's right for you will be a test of will, determination, and patience, because the only diet that will work for you is the one that's 100% customized for you.

I've learned that everyone wants to fit into a diet mold; to have the ease of being "gluten-free," "dairy-free," keto, paleo, or vegetarian. But you are not a pastry. There is no mold for you to perfectly fit. The belief that you can heal your gut simply by excluding an entire food group is false. Even with a diagnosis like celiac disease, where you will need to forever cut gluten, I can promise you there will be something more you need to do; something else you'll need to remove or add to your diet. What, I don't know, because we are all different, and your diet solution will be 100% customized for you.

Figuring out what will work for you—and what doesn't—is critical to healing not just your gut, but your entire body. Because 70% or more of your immune system lies in your gut, the health of your digestion and gut bacteria is critical to your overall well-being. And what you eat (or don't eat) can also have a tremendous effect on your daily energy levels. The foods that fuel you and those that zap you of energy are different for everyone.

I am a self-described "food detective," and in order to find the ideal diet for your body, you'll need to become one, too. During this 21-day journey, you must pay attention to the food you choose to nourish your body and be cognizant of how it is affecting your health. This starts with choosing the most nutrient-dense, real food you can every single chance you have, and steering clear of preservatives, chemicals, and anything artificial. But for many, this will not be enough. You will also need to learn and understand which foods are not supporting your healing process. You may need an elimination diet or specific blood tests to determine this. The process can be a lot of work, but I can guarantee that until you learn to fill your body with proper nutrition, you will never fully heal. Just like life, what we put in is what we get out.

LEAKY GUT SYNDROME

Leaky gut syndrome is at the top of many gut-related conversations and controversies these days. *Time* magazine recently published an article noting that research is beginning to validate the syndrome's existence: "So-called 'leaky gut syndrome' is legit, and likely plays a role in food allergies, type-1 diabetes, celiac disease, Crohn's disease, irritable bowel syndrome and other digestion-related maladies."[1] But there are many other doctors who believe there is no such thing as leaky gut syndrome, and suggest it is a "fad" rather than a real diagnosis. Former National Council Against Health Fraud president Robert S. Baratz, DDS, MD, PhD, claims, "Some fad diagnoses seem almost to be interchangeable. Large numbers of people are scammed in the same way for different conditions, by a variety of practitioners and unlicensed personnel. It is as though there is a 'menu' of quack treatments that they can choose for a variety of alleged conditions depending on the patient's susceptibility and pocketbook and the practitioner's guile, gall, and greed."[2]

Based on my own research and life experiences, I would have to fully disagree with Dr. Baratz. In 2009, I did a food intolerance test and the results showed that I was intolerant to 22 different foods, including egg whites, milk, shrimp, lentils, malt, and celery. There was no rhyme or reason to the list, but I worked very hard at avoiding all of them. What I would go on to learn in the years that followed was that I wasn't necessarily intolerant to all of those foods. Instead, my gut had become leaky, which was causing my body to react to those foods and so many more.

In the simplest terms, leaky gut syndrome is when the cells that make up the lining of the intestinal tract become so inflamed that the gut lining becomes more permeable than it's meant to be. (Note: many Western doctors prefer the term "intestinal permeability" to "leaky gut

---

[1] http://time.com/4178015/leaky-gut-syndrome-probiotics/
[2] http://www.quackwatch.com/01QuackeryRelatedTopics/fad.html

syndrome.") This can eventually result in "undigested food particles and gut flora enter[ing] the bloodstream."[3]

The symptoms of leaky gut syndrome can include any or all of the following:

1. Gas, bloating, constipation, diarrhea, or a combination
2. Seasonal allergies or asthma
3. Hormonal imbalances
4. An autoimmune disease
5. Chronic fatigue syndrome or fibromyalgia
6. Mood and mind issues (ADD, ADHD, etc.)
7. Skins issues like acne and rosacea
8. Candida overgrowth
9. Food allergies and intolerances
10. Inflammatory bowel disease (colitis, Crohn's, celiac, etc.)
11. Headaches

---

[3]http://www.organiclifestylemagazine.com/gluten-candida-leaky-gut-syndrome-and-autoimmune-diseases

So how do you get leaky gut syndrome? Those who believe it is a real syndrome mostly agree that it can be caused by various things that damage the gut in general, including:[4,5]

1. Alcohol and certain painkillers
2. Preexisting conditions like inflammatory bowel disease, gut infections, diabetes, complicated surgeries, and more
3. Sugar
4. Processed foods
5. Chronic stress
6. Toxins
7. Microbiome imbalance
8. Mold
9. Gluten

HOW TO FIX LEAKY GUT SYNDROME

If you accept the notion of leaky gut syndrome and believe it may be at the root of your own issues, here are some ways to fix it:

1. **Adjust your diet.** I recommend beginning with an elimination diet. While you can do food intolerance and allergy tests, if you actually do have a leaky gut, they may not be completely accurate. An elimination diet is the best way to identify which foods are irritating your gut. These will be different for everyone, but definitely begin by avoiding conventional dairy, sugar, gluten, chemicals, and other additives. Choose organic food whenever possible, and use caution with soy in particular—you may want to cut

---

[4]https://experiencelife.com/article/how-to-heal-a-leaky-gut/
[5]http://www.wellnessresources.com/health/articles/leaky_gut_syndrome_
   more_than_just_a_gut_problem/

out soy altogether for a while, but when reintroducing it, choose only organic and fermented soy products.

2. **Begin a food journal.** Track your daily food intake, mood, and overall feelings and look for patterns and progress from day to day.

3. **Eat the foods that will help rebuild your gut.** In particular, make sure you are getting enough omega-3s and, when the time is right, fermented foods. Bone broth is a great choice for leaky gut because it contains collagen and the amino acids proline and glycine, which can help heal damaged cell walls. I also recommend wild-caught fish, lemon, ginger, turmeric, teas, and especially coconut oil, whose fatty acids "are rich in antimicrobial properties that work fantastically well to decrease levels of bad yeast and bacteria in the gut (help say goodbye to candida and SIBO)."[6] Once your gut has sufficiently healed, eating a ton of fiber each day can also be helpful.

4. **Supplement.** You might need to supplement with things like digestive enzymes, glutamine, probiotics, licorice root, quercetin, methylsulfonylmethane (MSM), zinc, slippery elm, moringa, cod liver oil, hydrochloric acid (HCL), and more. Be aware that not all probiotics are created equal— they contain different strains, fillers, and ingredients, and the state of your gut will determine which is the right one for you. You can also feed your body prebiotics naturally with homemade kombucha and fermented veggies.

5. **Eat mindfully and without stress.** While it's important to look closely at your diet, stress can also play a large role in leaky gut syndrome. Try to avoid becoming obsessive over food and fitness.

---

[6]http://goodbyeleakygut.com/heal-leaky-gut-syndrome/

6. **Limit the use of alcohol and NSAIDs.** While I do enjoy a high-quality vodka water with lemon or lime every now and then, making it a rare occasion was essential to healing my gut.

7. **Choose medications wisely, and only take antibiotics when critical.** Proceed with caution on medications, and avoid antibiotics whenever possible. However, don't trust anyone who tells you they are *never* critical. Modern medicine is here for a reason, so if you absolutely need antibiotics or other medication, take it.

8. **Determine if you have an underlying condition or infection.** This means going to the doctor to get tests done (not Googling!). If you can, find yourself an amazing integrative medicine doctor.

9. **Reduce overall stress.** Be sure to get enough sleep, and in addition to cutting out toxic foods, you may also want to take a look at any toxic relationships or other lifestyle factors that are causing you stress.

Gut Healing Is Not a Diet—Or Maybe It Is

Changing your diet is so trendy these days. Everywhere you turn, someone is gluten-free, dairy-free, sugar-free, paleo, grain-free, egg-free, soy-free, or on some other "diet" bandwagon. My own past includes a major disordered eating pattern—I engaged in an insane fitness regimen and diet, which led to the demise of my hormones, gut, and overall well-being. Eventually, I realized that to begin healing, I'd need to change my relationship with food and allow myself to eat enough, without following a strict set of rules. Food no longer had any kind of power over me. When I wanted something, I had it. It was as simple as that.

I came to see "diet" as a nasty four-letter word. As it is true that gut healing is not a diet in the traditional sense of the word. When people think of diets, they almost automatically translate the word to *weight loss*. Real health and true gut healing never aim for weight loss. My 21-day plan is not a "crazy diet," and you will not automatically lose weight by following the Gutsy Girl way of eating. (Though it may naturally happen, as it does for 99% of my clients once they begin to heal.)

That said, I now fully believe that gut-healing is, in fact, a diet. It must be. But what I mean by this is simply that choosing the right food for your body requires a sense of commitment to *your* gut-healing process.

A "healthy diet" is subjective. What is healthy for one might not be for another. I can't tell you how many blogs, gut-healing websites, and medical publications I've read that say XYZ food is the best—always—for everyone, no matter what. These types of one-size-fits-all diets, though, never work. There are healing foods, and then there are foods that allow us to heal without making us miserable. I have learned over the last several years that there is a huge difference.

Here are a few general principles to keep in mind as you work toward finding the ideal diet to heal your own unique gut:

1. **Food source matters.** There is no such thing as processed garbage when eating for true healing. There is no magic food

packaged in the grocery store for you to conveniently pick up. A healing diet should be based on whole foods that have been minimally (if at all) processed. The closer to home and nature your food source is, the better.

2. **Learn to read labels.** If you don't care to be educated on labels and learn how to read them and understand ingredients, you might not be ready to heal your gut. Just because a label says "local ingredients," "natural," "organic," or anything else of the sort does *not* mean it actually is. During these 21 days (and as a great practice for life beyond the 21 days), you should pay careful attention to all labels. Familiarize yourself with as many ingredients and alternative names as possible.

3. **Home cookin' is a must.** You don't have to be Martha Stewart. You don't even have to love the kitchen, but you do have to figure out how to whip up the most very basic things on your own, at home in your own kitchen. It is shockingly surprising to me how many people don't know how to do this, or don't want to. McDonald's won't heal your gut . . . if you want to maintain control over what you're putting into your body, you need to learn to create it yourself.

4. **Drugs and medication may stall your progress.** While there is a place for medication in gut healing, and you should never quit cold turkey or without consulting your doctor, you need to know that drugs disrupt the gut flora. As long as you are dependent on drugs and drugs alone, you will likely never be healed. Even if you change your diet to heal your gut, if you consume a high quantity of medications your progress will probably be minimal.

5. **Let them eat cake.** Sure, your friends are posting pictures of their cake and ice cream, chips and cheese, Big Macs and whipped cream. They have found the best blogger who will show you how to make the most phenomenal-tasting,

low-budget meal with processed noodles, food colorings, and all sorts of other bright-colored, mouthwatering convenience items. Unfortunately, this is not the way to heal the gut. Let others eat their own cake . . . healing the gut has cake, too. (I've figured out various cake recipes that fit into my gut-healing diet, and you can do the same!)

6. **Cheating never works.** In order to figure out what foods work for you and which trigger your symptoms, you'll need to start with an elimination diet and then slowly add possible trigger foods back in, one by one. During the "elimination" phase, cheating is not allowed. In any trial period, the goal is to measure a certain set of criteria without disrupting the pattern. If the pattern is disrupted, the trial period ends because the results are skewed. In short, if you cheat, you will have to start over. It is these starts and stops that prohibit most people from ever healing their gut. If you won't hustle for your healthy lifestyle and healing your gut, then this method is not for you.

7. **Journaling will be your friend.** I'm not talking about journaling to keep track of every calorie and ounce of food you put in your body. But you will need a food journal where you can track several different things for a trial period of time to help determine which food and lifestyle factors are contributing to your problems. You can use the journaling pages in this book, my *Healing Blooms from Within* journal (see Resources, page 252), or any other notebook or digital journal you like. Don't want to make journaling a priority? You might not be ready to heal your gut.

8. **Where there is a will, there is a way.** Would you agree with me that excuses get old? Do you enjoy when your children give you excuses? Or your spouse? Or even friends and neighbors? If you're truly ready to heal your gut, you'll make no excuses, and you will forever be changed.

Finding *Your* Ideal Gutsy Girl Diet

If there's no one "right way" to eat, how do you go about finding the right diet for you? There are several different dietary changes you may need to consider, depending on your symptoms and diagnosis. For example, you might find you need to eliminate gluten, pay attention to FODMAPs, or create a plan that removes all dairy and dairy sources. You may need to combine several different strategies or pick and choose components from each one.

Here is a chart filled with various gut-healing diets as "templated plans" (see pages 49–51)." If any of them should strike a chord, you may want to discuss with your doctor or nutritionist how to make it work for you.

Say "Yes"

Figuring out the right diet for your own needs is a process, but the lists that follow are a good place to start when selecting gut-healthy, healing foods. Use the "Say Yes" list (see pages 54–55) as a jumping-off point as you embark on your 21-day journey, but remember that it is not meant to be an exhaustive list for what you *can* eat successfully. All the foods listed here have worked well for my individual and group program clients, but we are all so different, and some of these foods may be problematic for you. Listen to your body. If you suspect a food on the "Say Yes" list is giving you problems, remove it for 72 hours, then try it again. You might find your answers by doing that alone.

Fats and Oils: Please do not be fat phobic. Fat alone does not make us fat, and eating healthy fats from oils, raw nuts, and seeds *in moderation* can be very healing and therapeutic. They can also add a ton of natural flavor to meals. You may need to soak raw nuts and seeds prior to eating or eat nuts in raw nut butter form (as long as there are no additives). Fats and oils can be hard if you are struggling with diarrhea, so use nuts only in flour form until diarrhea has cleared. If you are constipated, however, these fats can help speed things along. Keep meticulous notes in your journal to identify patterns.

Nut-based flours like almond flour, almond meal, and coconut flour can be a good replacement for gluten- and grain-based flours. There is a huge

continued on page 53

GUT-HEALING DIETS

DIET TYPE	WHAT IT IS	WHO MAY BENEFIT
Autoimmune Protocol (AIP)[1]	This was originally developed by Loren Cordain, PhD, and popularized by Sarah Ballantyne, PhD. You must avoid processed foods, refined oils and sugars, grains and pseudo-grains (like quinoa), gluten, legumes, soy, dairy, nightshades, nonnutritive sweeteners (like stevia), eggs, nuts, seeds, and alcohol. There is a 30-day elimination period, and then you begin reintroducing things.	Those with an autoimmune condition
Anti-Inflammatory Diet	Low sugar, emphasis on fish over meat, healthy oils, and fats. Focused on reducing inflammation that may cause weight gain and health problems.	Anyone with suspected inflammation
Carnivore Diet	Eat meat, fish, eggs, and some dairy.	Those who cannot tolerate any sugars, carbs, fiber, or the like
Dairy-Free Diet	Consume nothing that contains dairy or its by-products.	Those with a dairy allergy and/or intolerance
Egg-Free Diet	Consume nothing that contains eggs or their by-products.	Those with an egg allergy and/or intolerance
Elimination Diet	An elimination diet involves removing "suspect" foods, and then later reintroducing them, one at a time. Simultaneously, you'll watch for symptoms that show a reaction.	Those who are stuck on what foods are truly aggravating symptoms and manifestations
Gluten-Free Diet	Consume nothing that contains gluten or its by-products.	Those with a gluten allergy and/or intolerance. Those with a confirmed celiac diagnosis
Glycemic Index (G.I.) Diet	Choose foods that are low on the glycemic index, which measures how quickly foods are digested.	Those with blood sugar problems

[1]https://www.amazon.com/gp/product/1936608391/ref=as_li_qf_sp_asin_il_tl?ie=UTF8&tag=agugi-20&camp=1789&creative=9325&linkCode=as2&creativeASIN=1936608391&linkId=a5ab33f9023125e949da26bcade8cd2d

GUT-HEALING DIETS (CONTINUED)

DIET TYPE	WHAT IT IS	WHO MAY BENEFIT
Gut and Psychology Syndrome (GAPS Diet)	Created by Natasha Campbell-McBride. Avoid processed foods, refined oils and sugars, grains, gluten, some lentils, soy. But you're still allowed to have things like nuts, peanuts, some sweeteners, some dairy (in fact, it's encouraged). There is a lot of emphasis on bone broth and fermented foods.	An intense gut-healing protocol for those who are open to certain dairy products, broth, and fermented foods
High-Fiber Diet[2]	Plant-based plan that challenges popular keto and paleo diets.	Those who need a plan for increasing fiber
Keto Diet	High fat, moderate protein, very low carb.	Those wishing to achieve ketosis
Leaky Gut Diet	A diet that promotes digestive health and focuses on vegetables, fruits, fermented vegetables, cultured dairy products, healthy fats, and lean, unprocessed meats. It moves through phases of elimination and then reintroduction.	Those with diagnosed or suspected leaky gut who want to go through phases of eliminating and then adding foods back in for gut health
Lectin-Free Diet	Eliminate foods that contain lectin, a plant protein that may be connected to inflammation in the body.	Those who have been told they cannot tolerate or process lectin-containing foods appropriately
Low-FODMAP Diet	The low-FODMAP diet is paying attention to the classification of foods known as FODMAPs. FODMAP stands for "fermentable oligosaccharides, disaccharides, monosaccharides, and polyols," which are short-chain carbohydrates and sugar alcohols that are poorly absorbed by the body. If and when they are poorly absorbed, abdominal pain and bloating can surface.	Diagnosed IBS and/or confirmed SIBO
Low-Histamine Diet[3]	Follow a diet which is low in histamine. Foods to avoid include things like fermented foods, wine, leftover meat, citrus fruits, most berries, and eggs.	Those with a histamine intolerance

---

[2]*Fiber Fueled: The Plant-Based Gut Health Program for Losing Weight, Restoring Your Health, and Optimizing Your Microbiome,* Dr. Will Bulsiewicz
[3]*The 4-Phase Histamine Reset Plan: Getting to the Root of Migraines, Eczema, Vertigo, Allergies and More,* Dr. Becky Campbell

GUT-HEALING DIETS (CONTINUED)

DIET TYPE	WHAT IT IS	WHO MAY BENEFIT
Mediterranean Diet	Plant, not meat-based; healthy fats are prioritized. Daily consumption of vegetables, fruits, and whole grains. Includes a variety of foods that build a stronger microbiome.	Those looking for overall health and/or a plan that's void of meat
Mold-Free Diet[4]	The idea is that molds are everywhere and are disrupting the microbiome for those with mold illness. The four categories of food to exclude on this diet include gluten, acellular carbohydrates (e.g., dried grains and seeds, flours, pulverized and liquid forms of starches and sugar, which are more present in the modern world diets) and refined sugar, dairy, and industrial seed oils.	Those with mold issues and/or symptoms pointing to a mold problem
Paleo Diet	Eat like a caveman, focusing on lean meats and fish, nuts and seeds, fruits and vegetables. Avoid dairy, sugar, legumes, and grains.	The backbone for many "gut-healing" diets.
Soy-Free Diet	Consume nothing that contains soy or its by-products.	Those with a soy allergy or intolerance
Specific Carbohydrate Diet (SCD)	This diet was created by Dr. Sidney Haas, but popularized by Elaine Gottschall. SCD is "based on the theory that by eliminating most carbs (primarily grains, starches, dairy, and sugars) and allowing only specific carbs that require minimal digestion, it can reduce inflammation and make eating enjoyable for people with gastrointestinal (GI) disorders."[5] On the diet, you should avoid all grains, beans, legumes, sugar, most dairy, starchy vegetables and non-grain flours, fermented beverages, and even chocolate/cacao.	Strict gut-healing protocol for those with a variety of GI problems
Vegan Diet	Eat only plant-based foods, including omitting anything that has any connection to animals, such as eggs, milk, or gelatin.	Those wishing to heal by way of consuming no animal products

[4]https://chriskresser.com/food-for-mold-illness-what-to-eat-and-what-to-avoid/
[5]https://elanaspantry.com/specific-carbohydrate-diet/

IS FIBER HELPING OR HURTING ME?

If you live with IBS and/or IBD, you may have heard a lot of conflicting information around eating fiber. Fiber is *phenomenal* for those without gut imbalances, which is why doctors recommend eating more of it for better digestion. It helps to slow digestion down, which explains why weight-loss gurus recommend it to help people stay fuller for longer.

But if you have IBD/IBS-C *and* slow motility, more fiber is probably not the answer for you.

And those with compromised guts should be aware that fiber is one of the natural habitats for bacteria in the gut. In fact, they feed on it. So fiber can ultimately provide a good habitat for the bad bacteria that are causing you discomfort, aggravating the inflammation in the gut wall.

Of course, fibrous foods are packed with nutrients that your body needs. But you *don't* need to eat those foods to get them.

One of the best ways to get all the nutritional benefits of fiber-rich fruits and veggies with none of the fiber-related issues is by juicing. Juicing removes the fiber, "which impairs absorption of many nutrients in fruit and vegetables and aggravates the condition in the already sensitive digestive system. The digestive system has virtually no work to do in digesting juices, they get absorbed in 20–25 minutes, providing the body with a concentrated amount of nutrients."[1] You can also try consuming foods that are high-fiber and low in FODMAPs to increase your fiber intake without aggravating your gut.

Just remember, no fiber at all is *not* an optimal solution for gut health.

---

[1] *Gut and Psychology Syndrome: Natural Treatment for Autism, Dyspraxia, A.D.D., Dyslexia, A.D.H.D., Depression, Schizophrenia*, by Dr. Natasha Campbell-McBride

difference between flours and meals, so be sure to use the right one for your recipe. I don't recommend a ton of nut flours and meals in the beginning of your healing process, though, as you may have adverse reactions to them for various reasons.

Ghee butter, while technically a dairy product, has had most of the lactose removed from it, so those who are unable to tolerate dairy tend to do very well with it. When using fish oil, never heat it, and make sure to choose a high-quality variety.

NOTE: Tree nuts like cashews, almonds, and walnuts are one of the major allergens. You likely already know if you are allergic to them, and if so, they are *definitely* not a "yes" food for you. I included them on this list because tree nuts make it possible to bake even when eating gluten-free, wheat-free, and grain-free. If you're allergic to tree nuts, though, you might need to skip baking for now.

Animal Proteins: I subscribe 100% to the theory that meat and poultry are not the enemy. Many of us have been taught to avoid these foods, but when we eat meat in its purest form, it can be very healing to the gut. It is, however, very important that you know where the meat came from. How was the animal raised? How was it fed? Choosing a high-quality meat *matters*. I don't eat a ton of meat anymore, but I include it in my diet when I can find grass-fed, organic, antibiotic-free meat.

Fruit: Fruits are packed full of vitamins and minerals and most of us love their sweet taste, but when the gut has been greatly compromised, they can be hard to digest. When you do choose to eat fruits, make sure they are fully ripened. This helps ensure they are easier to digest. For example, when a banana is very ripe, it is a monosaccharide, which tends to make it easier for the body to digest.

Your body will let you know which fruits you can and cannot handle, but the reality is that most, if not all, of the fruits listed here *could*

continued on page 56

"SAY YES" LIST

FATS/OILS

Almonds, raw

Almond Oil

Cashews, raw

Chia Seeds

Coconut Butter

Coconut Flour

Coconut Oil

Cod Liver Oil

Fish Oil

Ghee Butter

Hazelnuts, raw

Macadamia Nuts, raw

Nut Butters, made with raw nuts

Nut Flours, made with raw nuts

Olive Oil, cold pressed

Pecans, raw

Pumpkin Seeds

Sesame Seeds

Walnuts, raw

Walnut Oil, cold pressed

FISH

(wild-caught, never farmed)

Catfish

Cod

Flounder

Halibut

Mackerel

Pollock

Salmon

Sardine

Sole

Snapper

Trout

Tuna

FRUIT

Apple

Apricot

Avocado

Banana *(very ripe)*

Blackberry

Blueberry

Cherry

Coconut *(unsweetened, shredded)*

Kiwifruit

Lemon

Lime

Melon

Olive *(unprocessed, no added sulfites)*

Orange

Papaya *(ripe)*

Pear

Pineapple

Raspberry

Strawberry

HERBS/SPICES

Basil

Bay Leaf

Capers

Chamomile

Chervil

Chives

Cilantro

Cinnamon

Clove

Cumin

Dill

Garlic

Ginger

Lavender

Lemongrass

Marjoram

Mint

Mustard

Nutmeg

Oregano

Parsley

Pepper

Peppermint

Rosemary

Saffron

Sage

Salt *(sea or kosher)*

Spearmint

Tarragon

Thyme

Turmeric

LIQUIDS

Coconut Milk

Almond Milk

Water

Coffee

Tea

Broth (chicken, vegetable, and/or beef)

PANTRY INGREDIENTS

Baking Soda

Chia Seeds*

Flaxseed*

Hempseed*

Honey*

Maple Syrup

Mustard

Nutritional Yeast

Psyllium Husk*

Raisins/Dates (Medjool and California)*

Vanilla Extract

Vinegar

MEAT/POULTRY
(grass-fed, organic, and antibiotic-free when possible)

Beef

Bison

Buffalo

Chicken

Duck

Elk

Goose

Lamb

Organ Meat (such as liver)

Pheasant

Pork (which includes bacon, but it must be unprocessed and not contain sulfites)

Turkey

Veal

Venison

VEGETABLES

Acorn Squash*

Artichoke*

Arugula

Asparagus*

Bamboo Shoots

Beets*

Bok Choy

Broccoli*

Brussels Sprouts*

Butternut Squash*

Cabbage*

Cauliflower*

Celery*

Collard Greens

Cucumber (peeled and seeded)

Green Beans

Kale

Leek*

Lettuce (romaine, iceberg, green, red, butter)*

Mustard Greens

Onion*

Pumpkin*

Spinach

Spaghetti Squash*

Sweet Potato/Yam*

Swiss Chard

Water Chestnuts

Zucchini (peeled and seeded)

*Be cautious with the starred items. Keep meticulous notes in your journal to identify patterns.

present problems for you. Some, like apples, mangoes, and pears, are high in FODMAPs; berries like blackberries and strawberries may be too "seedy"; and others may present problems unique to *you*. Keep meticulous notes in your journal to identify patterns, and if raw, whole fruits cause issues for you, try eating them in juice and/or smoothie form, or on an empty stomach (not with other foods).

Vegetables: While vegetables are wonderful for us, they may make you miserable in the beginning of the healing process, mostly due to their fiber content. Many vegetables, like artichokes, asparagus, and broccoli, are also high in FODMAPs, which your body may not tolerate well. We want to get your digestive system back on track so that you can tolerate as many vegetables as possible. As you begin your 21-day journey, you will want to limit your vegetable intake to no more than ½ to ¾ cup per sitting. Be extra cautious of the starred items on the "Say Yes" list, and when you do consume them, be sure to keep diligent track of how your body reacts in your food journal.

The preparation can make a big difference when introducing more vegetables into your diet.

Steaming, for example, makes the vegetables softer and easier to digest. Before steaming veggies, prep them to make them as "digestive-system-friendly" as possible by removing skins and seeds. You can add flavor to steamed veggies by tossing in your favorite herbs and seasonings, squeezing fresh lemon juice over the top, or tossing with oil prior to eating.

Juicing is another great way to get more vegetables into your diet while healing. Juicing veggies helps remove most of the fiber and roughage that can aggravate gut-wall inflammation.

During my 101 days of intense gut healing, juicing was how I first introduced vegetables back into my diet. You may find success doing the same.

Herbs and Spices: Flavor, flavor, flavor: Herbs and spices add flavor to the Gutsy Girl's life. Not only that, but most have properties and benefits that can aid in your healing journey. Turmeric has been studied for its ability to reduce inflammation. Ginger has prokinetic abilities. In fact, almost every single common herb and spice has some gut-healing indication. Buy them in their whole, natural state and enjoy. Most herbs and spices will be okay in small doses, but keep meticulous track in case your gut doesn't do well with one or more of them.

Liquids: I swear by broth for helping to advance healing efforts. In fact, a South American proverb states, "Good broth will resurrect the dead." Whether or not you believe that, bone broth has been studied for benefits including boosting the immune system and helping to seal the intestinal lining (for leaky gut syndrome), and it is a nutrient-dense food. Make it homemade as often as possible.

Nut- and coconut-based milks can be a great replacement for dairy milk, but it's important to avoid varieties that contain carrageenan and added sugars. Choose only pure coconut milk or coconut milk with nothing but water added. Stay away from store-bought varieties of almond milk unless you can find one that's free of carrageenan and sugar. For tea, choose unprocessed varieties, and try to avoid black tea in the beginning of the 21-day process.

The only gut-health protocol that prohibits coffee is the autoimmune (AI) protocol. If your gut is not massively damaged and you know that coffee will not cause an immediate diarrhea reaction, go ahead and feel free to enjoy one small, unprocessed, diluted cup of coffee per day during these 21 days. "Small" means four to six ounces (don't cheat!). Choose unflavored, organic coffee with no added chemicals, and ideally dilute it with plenty of homemade almond or other nut milk or coconut milk. Remember not to add sugar. If you really need a touch of sweetness, use honey or a hint of maple syrup. I drink coffee like this daily with zero bloat (and for the love of coffee, life, and staying sane, we can't give up everything!), but when it comes to coffee, as always, please make the best and most informed decision for *you*.

Pantry Ingredients: You will rarely ever see a recipe of mine use baking powder, which contains starch (usually cornstarch) to make it rise better.

Baking soda, however, doesn't contain starch and can work alone in baking recipes with the magic of other natural ingredients (such as lemon).

Raisins, dates, and honey will be your "dessert" as you start on this journey. Limit these to a tablespoon or less per day, and be sure to choose varieties with no additives, and organic if possible. Honey is the preferred sweetener choice for Gutsy Girls, and even honey might be too much for you if you are battling candida. (I am a huge fan of coconut sugar as well, but it should be added in a little bit later.) Although you should only use honey minimally at first, many can tolerate it well because it's a monosaccharide and contains natural digestive enzymes. In baking recipes, you can swap in ½ to ¾ cup of honey for each 1 cup of white sugar. Lower the oven temperature by 25 degrees since you don't want the honey to reach a high temperature. And always use raw and unfiltered varieties—honey as Mother Nature intended. If baking with vanilla extract or other extracts, make sure the ingredients list includes only alcohol and the flavor, such as "vanilla bean."

When it comes to condiments, mustard is fine, if you carefully read the label. There should be no added sugars or other "Say No" ingredients. Use vinegars in small quantities only, and if you know you have a yeast overgrowth, avoid them altogether. Apple cider vinegar is the preferred type during these 21 days. You can also use red or white, if there is nothing else added to it. Stay away from balsamic vinegar if you have any known (or suspected) issues with mold.

I have seen conflicting information about nutritional yeast (some say it is "a gluten cross-reactor"), but I've tested it out for myself, and I do just fine with it. Of course, you might not, but generally, nutritional yeast is probably okay to enjoy.

Say "No"

At the start of your 21-day healing journey, you will need to eliminate all the foods that may be contributing to your gut issues. Your own elimination diet may vary depending on your unique diagnosis and symptoms, but the lists below offer a good starting point for you to discuss with your healthcare provider.

As with the "Say Yes" list, the "Say No" list (see pages 62–72) is not meant to be exhaustive—there may be foods not included here that you'll need to avoid due to an allergy or intolerance (such as a true food allergy to strawberries, for example), and as you begin to heal, you may find that you can gradually and carefully incorporate some of the foods listed here back into your diet. It's important to note that many ingredients will appear on food labels under a variety of different names. The lists that follow include all the different synonyms and alternate names for these ingredients, and the many sources in which you may find them. It is also very important to note that not all the sources listed under each category will *always* contain that ingredient. For example, not all candy contains gluten—but it often does, and you need to know all the possibilities. Furthermore, even if a certain type of candy does *not* contain gluten, it still contains something that should definitely be avoided for these 21 days.

Corn: Many people react to corn and/or corn products. Corn is a grain. You know that whole-kernel corn is corn, but the truth is that corn is hidden almost everywhere. Read product labels carefully and say "no" to corn during these 21 days.

Dairy: Unless you have a severe dairy intolerance or allergy, you can use ghee butter (see page 75), but say "no" to all other dairy during these 21 days. That said, I do believe in the power of raw dairy to help heal the gut (this topic could fill an entire book of its own!). If, after a few weeks, you can get your hands on any raw dairy, I'd recommend it.

Eggs: Eggs are a top allergen. Most people will be able to add them back in just fine, but if you really want to know, leave them out for the full 21 days. Typically, those who don't tolerate eggs well are only intolerant to the egg white, not the egg yolk. Pure egg yolk can be very healing, so if you want to include yolks only after a week or two, give it a try. Egg whites are mucus forming, and thus can be hard to digest. Once the gut has healed, though, whole eggs typically present no long-term problems.

In baking recipes, there are several substitutes you can use in place of eggs:

- **Ground Flaxseed or Chia Seeds:** 1 Tbsp. ground flaxseed or chia seeds + 3 Tbsp. water = 1 egg (Combine ingredients and whip by hand. Let the mixture sit for at least a few minutes before using.)
- **Applesauce:** ¼ cup unsweetened applesauce = 1 egg (This won't always be the perfect binder, but it will work in some recipes, especially those you want to be moist.)
- **Banana:** ½ ripe banana, mashed = 1 egg (Almost never does an "egg substitute" work when baking with coconut flour.)

Fish: All the items listed here are shellfish or contain shellfish. Shellfish are a top allergen, but you likely already know if you are allergic to them. For those who are not allergic, all of these may be perfectly fine to consume, but proceed with caution. I am not allergic to shellfish, and I consumed a variety of fish while healing. If you don't feel that you need to exclude these, you can move them to the "Say Yes" list.

Legumes & Beans: You know the old saying: "Beans, beans, the magical fruit . . . the more you eat, the more you toot." If your digestive system is trying to heal, these should be kept out of your diet (or greatly reduced) *temporarily.* (This does not include green beans.) To be clear, this is *just temporary.* See the Resources section (page 252) for more information on digesting beans.

Liquids: Avoid all liquids except those that are specifically included on the "Say Yes" list.

Meat: While grass-fed, organic, antibiotic-free fresh meat is fine during these 21 days, you'll find a number of other meat forms you should avoid listed under various other categories above. For example, hot dogs are to be avoided because they usually contain wheat or gluten. Be sure to avoid all processed meats, as well as any meats from animals treated with antibiotics. Remember, we are what we eat.

Molds: If you have persistent irritable bowel symptoms, you might have mold sensitivity as well, which can be aggravated by foods that contain mold spores and other fungi. In addition to the items listed here, fruit is another ingredient that is prone to mold growth, which is another reason that for these first 21 days, I think it's best to limit the amount of fruit you eat per day. Eating too much fruit can contribute to candida overgrowth. But I do not think that most people need to completely remove fruit from their diets. Choose appropriate fruits that are listed on the "Say Yes" list, and keep your fruit as fresh as possible to avoid mold growth.

Nightshades: Nightshades can have huge negative implications for those who are already experiencing inflammation throughout the body. I have only included the nightshades you are likely currently eating on the list below. I did not include things like tobacco, but you should know that it is also a nightshade. All types of white and red potatoes are included on this list, but fortunately sweet potatoes are not!

Processed Food & Fast Food: Say "no" to anything processed. This could be your most difficult challenge during these 21 days, but it's necessary. Processing food strips it of anything that could potentially be good for us, and instead turns it into something that continues to wreak havoc on the digestive system. If it's packaged and processed with ingredients you can't possibly pronounce, don't buy it. If you need to go through a drive-through to obtain it, turn that car right around! Many of the foods on the "no" list are processed. For a simple definition of "processed foods," see the Glossary on page 264.

"SAY NO" LIST

One of the hardest parts of any food elimination diet is learning to decode labels and figure out where common trigger ingredients may be hiding out of sight. The lists below include common sources and alternate names for the foods you should be saying "no" to during these next 21 days.

CORN[1]

Acetic Acid

Alcohol

Alpha Tocopheral

Artificial Flavoring

Artificial Sweetener

Ascorbate

Ascorbic Acid (*Vitamin C*)*

Aspartame

Baking Powder

Blended Sugar

Cake

Calcium Citrate

Calcium Fumarate

Calcium Gluconate

Calcium Lactate

Calcium Stearate

Caramel

Caramel Coloring

Candy

Canned Fruit

Cellulose Microcrystalline

Cereal

Citrus Cloud Emulsion

Confectioners' Sugar

Cookies

Corn

Corn Alcohol

Corn Gluten

Corn Extract

Cornflour

Cornmeal

Cornstarch

Corn Oil

Corn Oil Margarine

Corn Sweetener

Corn Sugar

Corn Syrup

Corn Syrup Solids

Crystalline Dextrose

Crystalline Fructose

Dextrin

Dextrose

D-Gluconic Acid

Distilled White Vinegar

Erythritol

Ethanol

Ferrous Gluconate

Flavorings

Food Starch

Fructose

Fruit Juice Concentrate

Gluconate

Glucose

Glucose Syrup

Glutamate

Gluten

Glycerides

Golden Syrup

Gravy

Grits

High-Fructose Corn Syrup (*HFCS, HFCS 42, HFCS 55*)

Hominy

Hydrolyzed Corn

Hydrolyzed Corn Protein

Hydrolyzed Vegetable Protein

Ice Cream

Infant Formula (*in case you have an infant*)

Inositol

Invert Sugar

Invert Syrup

Iodized Salt

Jam

Jelly

[1]https://agutsygirl.com/2015/01/23/134-corn-sources-and-alternate-names/
*Even though this is listed under corn, you can take it as a supplement, if you need it.

Ketchup

Lactate

Lactic Acid

Lauryl Glucoside

Lecithin

Linoleic Acid

Lysine

Maize

Malt

Malt Extract

Malt Syrup

Maltitol

Maltodextrin

Maltose

Mannitol

Masa Harina

Mayonnaise

Methyl Glucose

Modified Cellulose Gum

Modified Cornstarch

Modified Food Starch

Molasses

Monosodium Glutamate

MSG

Natural Flavorings

Olestra/Olean

Polenta

Polydextrose

Polysorbates (e.g., Polysorbate 80)

Popcorn

Potassium Citrate

Potassium Gluconate

Powdered Cellulose

Powdered Sugar

Processed Food

Pudding

Saccharin

Salad Dressing

Semolina

Soda

Sodium Citrate

Sodium Erythorbate

Sodium Starch Glycolate

Sorbate

Sorbic Acid

Sorbitan

Sorbitol

Splenda

Starch

Stearic Acid

Sucralose

Sucrose

Sugar

Sweet'N Low

Syrup

Unmodified Starch

Vegetable Gum Protein

Vegetable Paste

Vegetable Starch

Xanthan Gum

Xylitol

Yeast

Zea Mays

"SAY NO" LIST (continued)

DAIRY[2]

Acidophilus Milk

Acid Whey

Ammonium Caseinate

Artificial Butter Flavor

Butter (*ghee butter is allowed, unless you have a severe dairy intolerance/ allergy*)

Butter Extract

Butter Fat

Butter-Flavored Oil

Buttermilk (*or buttermilk solids*)

Buttermilk Blend

Calcium Caseinate

Casein

Casein Hydrolysate

Caseinate

Cheese

Cheese Flavor

Condensed Milk

Cottage Cheese

Cream

Cream Cheese

Cultured Milk

Curds

Cured Whey

Custard

Dairy Product Solids

Delactosed Whey

Demineralized Whey

Diacetyl

Dried Milk

Dried Milk Solids (*DMS*)

Evaporated Milk

Galactose

Gelato

Goat's Milk

Half & Half

Hydrolyzed Casein

Hydrolyzed Whey

Ice Cream

Ice Milk

Imitation Cheese

Imitation Sour Cream

Iron Caseinate

Kefir

Lactaid® Milk

Lactalbumin

Lactalbumin Phosphate

Lactate Solids

Lactitol Monohydrate

Lactoglobulin

Lactose

Lactulose

Lactic Yeast

Magnesium Caseinate

Malted Milk

Margarine

Milk (*1% milk, 2% milk, low-fat milk, fat-free milk, full-cream milk, nonfat milk, nonfat dry milk, skim milk, whole milk*)

Milk Derivative

Milk Fat

Milk Powder

Milk Protein Hydrolysate

Milk Solids

Milk Solid Pastes

Natural Butter

Natural Butter Flavor

Nisin Preparation

Nonfat Milk Solids

Nougat

Pasteurized Milk

Potassium Caseinate

Powdered Milk

Powdered Whey

Pre-Made Soups and Sauces

Protein Hydrolysate

Pudding

Quark

Recaldent

Reduced Mineral Whey

Rennet

Rennet Casein

Sheep's Milk

Skim Milk Powder

Sodium Caseinate

[2]https://agutsygirl.com/2015/04/12/100-dairy-sources-alternate-names/

Sour Cream

Sour Cream Solids

Sour Milk

Sour Milk Solids

Sweet Cream Buttermilk Powder

Sweet Dairy Whey

Sweetened Condensed Milk

Tagatose

Vegetarian Cheeses with Casein

Whey

Whey Hydrolysate

Whey Protein Concentrate

Whey Powder

Whey Protein Hydrolysate

Whey Solids

Whipped Cream

Yogurt

Yogurt Powder

Zinc Caseinate

EGGS[3]

Aioli

Albumin

Apovitellin

Baked Goods

Bread

Breaded Food

Cake

Candy

Casserole

Conalbumin

Cookies

Croissant

Custard

Dried Egg

Dried Egg Solids

E-161b

Egg Beaters

Egg Protein

Egg Wash

Egg White

Egg Yolk

Eggnog

Energy Bars

Globulin

Hollandaise Sauce

Ice Cream

Livetin

Lysozyme

Mayonnaise

Meringue

Muffin

Ovalbumin

Ovoglobulin

Ovomucin

Ovomucoid

Ovotransferrin

Ovovitellin

Pancake

Pastry

Powdered Egg

Protein Powder

Protein Shakes

Pudding

Punch Egg

Quiche

Rolls

Silici Albuminate

Simplesse

Surimi

Tartar Sauce

Trailblazer

Vitellin

[3]https://agutsygirl.com/2015/11/15/52-egg-sources-and-alternate-names/

"SAY NO" LIST (continued)

FISH

Abalone	Escargot	Quahog
Anchovy	Fish Sauce	Roe
Barnacle	Fish Stock	Scallop
Bouillabaisse	Jambalaya	Scampi
Caesar Salad Dressing	Krill	Sea Cucumber
Calamari	Limpet	Sea Urchin
Caponata	Littleneck	Seafood Flavoring
Caviar	Lobster	Shrimp
Clam	Marinara Sauce	Snail
Cherrystone	Mollusks	Squid
Cockle	Mussel	Surimi
Crab	Octopus	Turban Shell
Crab Cake	Oyster	Whelk
Crawdads	Periwinkle	Worcestershire Sauce
Crawfish	Pismo	
Crayfish	Prawns	

LEGUMES & BEANS[4]

Acacia	Cape Gum	Green Bean (almost always, on every single gut-healing protocol, green beans are perfectly fine to consume during the 21 days)
Adzuki Bean	Carob	
Alfalfa	Chickpea	
Anasazi Bean	Cowpea	
Asparagus Bean	Dwarf Pea	
Astragalus	English Pea	Green Pea
Baked Beans	Falafel	Gum Arabic
Bean Sprouts	Farinata	Hummus
Berbera Gum	Fava Bean	Indian Gum
Black Bean	Field Pea	Java Bean
Blackeyed Pea	Garbanzo Bean	Kidney Bean
Butter Bean	Gram Flour	Lentil

[4]https://agutsygirl.com/2017/03/03/53-legume-and-bean-sources-and-alternate-names/

Licorice

Lima Bean

Locust Bean Gum

Masur Bean

Mongo Bean

Mung Bean

Mung Dal

Navy Bean

Peanut Butter

Peanut

Pink Bean

Pinto Bean

Red Bean

Snow Pea

Southern Pea

Soy

Soybean

String Bean

Sugar Snap Pea

Wax Bean

White Bean

LIQUIDS

Alcohol

Packaged Juices, Energy Drinks, etc.

Soda

MOLDS*

Beer

Black Tea

Bread

Cheese

Chocolate

Fruit Juice

Grains

Jam

Jelly

Malted Grain

Miso

Mushroom

Peanut

Pistachio

Vinegar

Wine

NIGHTSHADES

Ashwagandha

Bell Pepper

Cape Gooseberry (also known as ground cherries; not to be confused with regular cherries)

Cayenne Pepper

Chili Pepper

Chili Powder

Curry Powder

Eggplant

Garden Huckleberry

Goji Berry

Hot Pepper

Jalapeño Pepper

Ketchup

Marinara

Naranjilla

Paprika

Pimento

Potato (white and red, not sweet potato)

Red Pepper

Tobacco (chewing and smoking)

Tomatillo

Tomato Sauce

Tomato

* There are items on this list that are included in the Creations (mushrooms, pistachios, vinegar, etc.). If molds are not problematic for you, they do not need to be on the "Say No" list. If you're unsure, just be sure to meticulously track in your journal.

"SAY NO" LIST (continued)

SOY[5]

Artificial Flavoring	MSG	Soy Protein Isolate
Bean Curd	Natto	Soy Sauce
Bread	Natural Flavoring	Soy Sprouts
Bouillon Cubes	Non-Dairy Creamer	Soya Flour
Bulking Agent	Nimame	Soya
Candy	Okara	Soybean Curd
Carob	Processed Food	Soybean Flour
Cereal	Protein Powder	Soybean Granules
Chicken Broth (packaged)	Shirataki Noodles	Soybean Paste
Chocolate	Shoyu Sauce	Soybeans
Coffee Substitute	Soja	Supro
Deli Meat	Soy Albumin	Tamari
Edamame	Soy Bran	Tempeh
Energy Bar	Soy Concentrate	Teriyaki Sauce
Glycerin	Soy Cheese	Textured Soy Flour
Gravy	Soy Fiber	Textured Soy Protein
Gum Arabic	Soy Flour	Textured Vegetable Protein (TVP)
Hydrolyzed Soy Protein	Soy Lecithin	Tofu
Kinako	Soy Milk	Vegetable Broth (packaged)
Kinnoko Flour	Soy Oil	Vegetable Gum
Kyodofu	Soy Grits	Vegetable Starch
Margarine	Soy Nuts	Yakidofu
Mayonnaise	Soy Nut Butter	Yuba
Miso	Soy Protein	
Mono-Diglyceride	Soy Protein Concentrate	

NOTE: Some soy products can actually be very good for us (i.e., fermented soy like miso and tempeh). During this trial period, opt to leave it out.

[5]https://agutsygirl.com/2019/05/06/73-soy-sources-and-alternate-names/

SUGAR[6]

Acesulfame-K

Agave Nectar

Agave Syrup

Amasake

Amber Liquid Sugar

Apple Sugar

Apply Syrup

Arenga Sugar

Aspartame

Bakers Special Sugar

Barbados Sugar

Barley Malt

Barley Malt Syrup

Bar Sugar

Beet Molasses

Beet Sugar

Beet Syrup

Berry Sugar

Blackstrap Molasses

Brown Rice Syrup

Brown Sugar

Buttery Syrup

Cake

Cane Crystals

Cane Juice (evaporated)

Cane Juice Crystals

Cane Juice Powder

Cane Sugar

Caramel

Carob Syrup

Castor Sugar

Cellobiose

Chicory

Coarse Sugar

Coco Sugar

Coconut Nectar

Coconut Sugar (coconut palm sugar)*

Concord Grape Juice Concentrate

Confectioners' Sugar

Cookies

Corn Sweetener

Cornsweet 90

Corn Syrup

Corn Syrup Solids

Creamed Honey (this is not the natural honey)

Crystal Dextrose

Crystalline Fructose

Crystallized Organic Cane Juice

D-Arabino-Hexulose

D-Fructose

D-Mannose

D-Xylose

Dark Brown Sugar

Dark Molasses

Date Sugar

Decorating Sugar

Dehydrated Sugarcane Juice

Demerara Sugar

Dextran

Dextrin

Dextrose

Diastatic Malt

Diatase

Dixie Crystals

ECJ

Equal

Erythritol (alcohol)

Ethyl Maltol

First Molasses

Florida Crystals

Fructamyl

Fructose

Fruit Juice

Fruit Juice Concentrate

Galactose

Glucomalt

Glucoplus

Glucose

Glucose Solids

Glucose Sweet

Glucose Syrup

Glycol (alcohol)

Golden Syrup

Gomme Syrup

Granulated Fructose

Granulated Sugar

[6]https://agutsygirl.com/2014/06/10/192-sugar-sources-and-alternate-names/

"SAY NO" LIST (continued)

Granulated Sugarcane Juice

Grape Sugar

Gum

Gur

High-Dextrose Glucose Syrup

High-Fructose Corn Syrup (HFCS, HFCS 42, HFCS 55)

High-Fructose Maize Syrup

High-Maltose Corn Syrup

HSH

Hydrogenated Starch

Hydrogenated Starch Hydrosylate

Hydrolyzed Cornstarch

Icing Sugar

Inulin

Inverted Sugar Syrup

Invert Syrup

Isoglucose

Isomalt

Jaggery

Lactitol

Lactose

Levulose

Light Brown Sugar

Light Molasses

Liquid Sugar

Malt

Malt Syrup

Malted Barley Syrup

Malted Corn Syrup

Maltitol

Maltitol Syrup

Maltodextrin

Maltose

Mannitol (alcohol)

Maple Sugar

Maple Syrup (Can choose a hint of this, if needed.)

Meritose

Meritab 700

Mints

Misri

Monkfruit*

Mycose

Mylose

Nutra-sweet

Organic Agave Syrup

Organic Brown Rice Syrup

Organic Raw Sugar

Organic Sucanat

Organic Sugar

Orgeat Syrup

Pancake Syrup

Panela

Panocha

Pearl Sugar

Powdered Sugar

Pure Cane Syrup

Pure Sugar Spun

Raisin Syrup

Raffinose

Rapadura

Raw Agave Syrup

Raw Sugar

Refiner's Syrup

Rice Malt

Rice Syrup

Rice Syrup Solids

Rock Sugar

Saccharin

Saccharose

Sanding Sugar

Shakar

Simple Syrup

Sirodex

Sorbitol (alcohol)

Sorghum

Sorghum Syrup

Splenda

Sucrose

Sucrosweet

Sugar

Sugar Beet Crystals

Sugar Beet Syrup

Sugarcane Juice

Sugarcane Natural

Sulfured Molasses

Sweet'N Low

Sweetened Condensed Milk

Sweetleaf

Table Sugar

Tagatose

Treacle

Triose

Truvia

Turbinado Sugar

Unrefined Sugar

White Crystal Sugar

White Grape Juice Concentrate

White Refined Sugar

White Sugar

Wood Sugar

Xylose

Xylitol (alcohol)

Yellow Sugar

* I use coconut sugar frequently in many different things, in cooking and in baking. You will notice it from several of my recipes. For the 21 days, though, I recommend leaving it out.

* I do use monkfruit occasionally now, with no side effects. For the 21 days I recommend leaving it out, but then feel free to experiment with it.

WHEAT AND GLUTEN[7]

Ale

All-Purpose Flour

Artificial Flavor/Artificial Flavoring

Atta

Barley

Beer

Bouillon Cubes

Bran

Bread

Bread Crumbs

Bread Stuffing

Breaded/Battered Foods

Brewer's Yeast

Broth

Brown Flour

Bulgur

Cake

Candy

Cereal

Coffee and Tea (flavored)

Cookies

Couscous

Cracked Wheat

Crackers

Deli Meat

Dinkel

Dumplings

Durum

Edible Starch

Einkorn

Emmer

Enriched Flour

Farina

Farro/Faro

Flour

Flour Tortillas

Fu

Germ

Gluten

Graham Flour

Granary Flour

Gravies and Sauces (thickened with flour)

Groats

Hard Wheat

Hing

Hordeum Vulgare

Hot Dog

Hydrolyzed Wheat Protein

Ice Cream Cones

Imitation Bacon Bits

Imitation Seafood (e.g., crab)

Kamut

Lager

Licorice

Lunch Meat (processed)

Macha Wheat

Maida

Malt

[7]https://agutsygirl.com/2016/04/11/124-wheat-and-gluten-sources-and-alternate-names/

"SAY NO" LIST (continued)

Malt Extract

Malt Flavoring

Malt Syrup

Malt Vinegar

Malted Milk

Marinade

Matzo

Matzo Meal

Meatloaf (typically made with bread crumbs)

Meripro 711

Mir

Modified Food Starch

Modified Wheat Starch

Muffins

Natural Flavor/Natural Flavoring

Nishasta

Noodles

Oats/Oatmeal

Oriental Wheat

Orzo

Pan Spray

Pasta

Pearl Barley

Persian Wheat

Perungayam

Pie Crust

Pita Bread

Polish Wheat

Poulard Wheat

Pretzels

Processed Foods

Rolled Oats

Roux

Rusk

Rye

Salad Dressing

Sauce

Sausage

Scotch

Seitan

Semonlina

Soup

Soup Base

Soy Sauce

Spelt

Stone-Ground Wheat

Stout

Strong Flour

Tabbouleh

Teriyaki Sauce

Textured Vegetable Protein–TVP

Triticale

Triticum Vulgare

Udon

Unbleached Flour

Vavilovi Wheat

Vegetable Starch

Wheat Berries

Wheat Bran

Wheat Flour

Wheat Germ

Wheat Starch

Whiskey

Soy: Soy is a top allergen. The way we have "Westernized" it has made it hard on the digestive system, and most soy is genetically modified. Some fermented soy products, like miso and tempeh, can actually be very good for us, but during this trial period, it's best to leave all soy out.

Sugar: Say "no" to sugar during these 21 days (except the carefully chosen natural sugars included in the "Say Yes" section on page 55). Remember that sugar can be found under many different labels. All added sugars must be cut, and it's best to limit even fruit during this time. All "natural" sugars, artificial sweeteners, and sugar alcohols must be avoided. (While stevia doesn't contain sugar, for example, it usually has many other added things to it that make it a No during these 21 days.)

Wheat and Gluten: Even if you do not have celiac disease, chances are that if you have IBS or IBD, you are sensitive to wheat and/or gluten, and you may experience symptoms of gluten sensitivity outside the gut as well. The bottom line is, during this time, you must avoid them. Note that I've categorized wheat and gluten together here, but they are *not* the same thing. Wheat is a grain. Gluten is a protein. If something says "gluten-free," then it's always wheat-free, but if something says "wheat-free," it's not necessarily gluten-free. That said, during your initial 21 days you won't need to worry about the difference, since you won't be eating either. While oats are technically gluten-free, you should generally avoid them because they are almost always processed in mills that process grains containing gluten. There are some brands that make them gluten-free now but stay away from even those during these 21 days.

MAKING GLUTEN-FREE A GAME

When you take a staple like gluten out of your diet, you may find yourself thinking, "Oh my God, I'm going to starve!" But life should be fun, and there's no reason going gluten-free needs to be so serious or frightening. To make it a little easier, I've found several ways to "gamify" the gluten-free lifestyle:

1. *Food Market Search.* Each time I go to the grocery store or farmers market, I try to buy one new gluten-free product I've never had before. It might be a new fruit, vegetable, or beverage, or a packaged item clearly labeled with the gluten-free tag. I've found some great ingredients this way I might otherwise never have tried. One year I picked up some moringa, and I never looked back!

2. *Gluten-Free Scavenger Hunt.* Do you have Google Maps on your phone? Of course you do. The next time you are out and about in an area you're not as familiar with, go to Google Maps and type "Gluten-Free" in the search bar, and then head to whatever restaurant or store you find. This game has led me to stumble upon some great new things, like a local pizzeria that carries a gluten-free crust. This game works equally well with Foursquare, Yelp, or any other location-based application. And as a bonus, you'll often find tips that previous reviewers have left to help you decide what to try.

3. *"Your New Favorite Blog" Search.* Do a Google search for "gluten-free blogs" and see what comes up. Add the ones that look promising to your Google Reader, bookmark them, or save them via a service like Bloglovin'. You'll get a ton of great ideas, and maybe even find a new favorite blog.

4. *Recipe Challenge.* Be the star of your own cooking show—create your own original recipe and see what happens! When I'm working on a new recipe, I like to start by making a list of all the ingredients I'm interested in using, cross-check to be sure they're gluten-free, and then start playing with different ways to combine and bring those ingredients to life. Use a cookbook, or better yet, don't, and see what you come up with.

Going gluten-free can seem hard and overwhelming in the beginning, but give it time, practice, explore, and throw in a bit of fun, and after a while it will become second nature to you.

WHAT IS GHEE BUTTER?

Ghee is simply butter that has been clarified, which means it has been melted over low heat for an extended period of time eliminating most of the moisture and cause the milk solids to caramelize. Once it's cooled, the top layer is skimmed off, and this layer of pure fat is the ghee. The process of cooking off the milk solids burns off most of the lactose found in normal butter. This makes ghee a great alternative to dairy butter for those who are lactose-intolerant. Ghee has a great slightly nutty taste and a long shelf life. It can last for several weeks in your pantry, or up to 6 months in the fridge. I recommend organic ghee butter from Organic Valley or 4th & Heart, both of which you can find at Amazon or Whole Foods.

Supplements

Dietary changes can go a long way toward healing your gut, but you may also want to address deficiencies in certain vitamins, minerals, and nutrients with the help of supplements. To avoid over (or under) supplementing, you *must* work with your practitioner. If the levels of nutrients in your body are too high or too low, it can throw off the body's natural function. In addition to being dangerous in some cases, at a bare minimum this can make your gut issues worse. However, when a supplement is recommended by your practitioner, try it.

Here are some supplements your practitioner might recommend for your healing journey.

*The brands with asterisks by them are brands I believe in so much so that not only do I use them, but they are *A Gutsy Girl* partners. Should you purchase directly from their website, you will save money just by using my code AGUTSYGIRL at checkout. You'll also find more brands, websites, and savings via the Resources section.

SUPPLEMENT	WHAT IT'S FOR	FAVE BRAND(S)
Adrenal Glandular	Gently nourishes adrenal glands to help overcome the effects of adrenal fatigue	Dr. Ron's Ultra Pure
Apple Cider Vinegar Complex	Reasons people use it: · Contains a small amount of magnesium, which helps with constipation. · The high level of acidity acts as a natural laxative by stimulating the colon into peristalsis (muscle contractions that move waste through the colon). · It contains natural probiotics, which may help with your immune system and gut health. · Contains acetic acid, and research shows that both acetic acid and butyric acid could relieve constipation.[8]	Paleovalley*

---

[8]https://www.sciencedirect.com/science/article/pii/S1756464620301778#:~:text
=And%20only%20the%20increase%20in,key%20roles%20in%20constipation%20
alleviation

Berberine	Berberine, typically used in conjunction with Allimax and Neem, helps support a healthy balance of microbes in the GI and respiratory tracts, and consists of a compound found in Oregon grape, barberry, goldenseal, and other herbs. It has been found that Berberine protects intestinal mucosal integrity.[9]	Thorne Research
Collagen	Collagen provides the amino acids needed to repair and rebuild the intestinal wall and prevent a leaky gut.	My Gut Garden*
Deglycyrrhizinated Licorice (DGL)	Deglycyrrhizinated licorice (DGL) helps your body repair your gut lining by replenishing the mucus that creates a healthy intestinal barrier.[10]	Pure Encapsulations
Digestive Enzymes	Support the breakdown, absorption, and utilization of macronutrients. Additionally, they help the body break down food and assist with optimal digestion.	My Gut Garden* Enzymedica—Digest Gold
Dysbiocide	Dysbiocide® supplies a proprietary blend of herbs and herbal extracts to support normal gut health. Select herbs get recognition for promoting the synergistic healing of damaged intestinal tissue, resulting predominately from dysbiosis. The combination of Eastern and Western herbs in this formula provides a broad anti-dysbiotic effect, even with low dosing.	Biotics Research Corporation
Epsom Salt	Epsom salt baths help with muscle relaxation, so if you struggle with constipation, an Epsom salt bath can help with movement. (Note: If you have diarrhea, you will *not* want to do this.)	N/A

---

[9] https://www.ncbi.nlm.nih.gov/pmc/articles/PMC5290458/
[10] https://www.amymyersmd.com/article/restore-gut-health-herbs-nutrients/

SUPPLEMENT	WHAT IT'S FOR	FAVE BRAND(S)
Gluten Away	Gluten Away is a unique blend of powerful digestive enzymes and probiotics designed to enhance optimal gluten digestion, protect against hidden sources of gluten, and support the complete digestion of gluten and other inflammatory wheat-derived peptides *within 60 to 90 minutes.* Taking this product isn't a license to consume gluten whenever and wherever. It's simply to help with unwanted gluten exposure.	Just Thrive Health*
Gut 4-tify	A supplement that helps seal and protect the mucosal barrier. Neutralizes free radicals before they can cause damage to the mucosal barrier. Delivers a patented citrus polyphenol extract that strengthens your gut barrier and maintains a balanced gut microbiome.	Just Thrive Health*
HCL	As the body ages, the amount of hydrochloric acid secreted to aid in digestion decreases. This leads to a condition known as hypochlorhydria. Hypochlorhydria begins as a gut deficiency and is one of the leading causes of gas and indigestion, and it can lead to many diseases and chronic inflammation. Without this important stomach acid, protein cannot be digested and many nutrients cannot be absorbed. In addition, acid from the stomach is a signal to the pancreas to perform its function, so hypochlorhydia can lead to problems in the pancreas as well. Diseases associated with low stomach acid include asthma, lupus, anemia, psoriasis, arthritis, ulcers, and many more. Indicators of low stomach acid can be simple gas and bloating, or more complex conditions, such as food allergies, constipation, anemia, and nausea.[11]	Integrative Therapeutics—Betaine HCL

---

[11] https://www.naturalnews.com/027979_digestive_enzymes_bloating.html#ixzz2HVugwhd6

SUPPLEMENT	WHAT IT'S FOR	FAVE BRAND(S)
Intestinal Movement Formula	If your doctor says, "Take Miralax," ask if you can try this instead. Acts as a natural laxative, non-habit-forming.	HealthForce Super Foods
ION Biome	Unfortunately, in our daily lives now we face the presence of potent toxins to these tight junctions, herbicides like Roundup, pharmaceuticals, refined gluten, etc. ION Biome supports the presence and integrity of these critical barrier systems.	ION Biome
L-glutamine	According to Dr. Josh Axe, glutamine is "an essential amino acid that is anti-inflammatory and necessary for the growth and repair of your intestinal lining. L-glutamine acts a protector and coats your cell walls, acting as a repellent to irritants."[12]	Now Foods 100% Pure— Free Form, powder version
Magnesium	Magnesium is a *macro* mineral that aids in everything from maintaining fluid balance to protecting metabolic health and supporting muscle and nerve function. It is critical for the Gutsy women with constipation.	Perfect Supplements*
Marshmallow Root	Dr. Josh Axe states, "Marshmallow helps restore integrity of the gut lining by forming a protective layer around small junctions. In addition, it seems to be beneficial for people suffering from other forms of inflammatory bowel diseases, including ulcerative colitis and Crohn's disease."[13]	N/A

---

[12]https://draxe.com/nutrition/l-glutamine-benefits-side-effects-dosage/#:~:text=Conclusion-,Glutamine%20is%20one%20of%2020%20naturally%20occurring%20amino%20acids%20found,to%20keep%20replenishing%20your%20supply
[13]https://draxe.com/nutrition/marshmallow-root/

SUPPLEMENT	WHAT IT'S FOR	FAVE BRAND(S)
Multivitamin	Make sure to get a quality one without any extra additives. A quality one *may* replace several individual vitamins.	Ortho Molecular Pure Encapsulations
N-acetylcysteine (NAC)	The effects of NAC are associated with some intestinal cell signaling pathways, such as EGFR, TLR4, apoptosis, and tight junction signaling.	N/A
Probiotic	An excellent probiotic is often a critical component for rebuilding healthy gut flora. Probiotics can help leaky gut by assisting in the maintenance of normal mucosa (gut wall lining) function and also protecting the lining from toxins, infections, and allergens. That said, too many probiotics in the beginning of the healing process can, for many people, contribute to the overpopulation of bad flora. Your circumstances will determine the probiotic species and strains you need.	Just Thrive Health*
Vitamin C	I take mine in powder form, but never in high doses. Vitamin C is critical for overall immune health, but it also helps prevent constipation.	Paleovalley Doctor's Best
Vitamin D	This is a nutrient most people are lacking, since the body needs sun to create it and many of us avoid the sun or wear sunscreen daily.	Perfect Supplements* Seeking Health
Zinc	Zinc is an essential trace mineral that is involved in numerous aspects of cellular metabolism. It is required for the catalytic activity of approximately 100 enzymes, and it plays a role in immune function, protein synthesis, wound healing, DNA synthesis, and cell division. It's also been shown that a zinc deficiency alters gut microbiota.[14]	Integrative Therapeutics Thorne Research Perfect Supplements*

---

[14] https://www.mdpi.com/2072-6643/7/12/5497

NOTE: I've said it before, but I must say it 10 million times: I am not a doctor. I am a Holistic Health Coach. I am not an expert when it comes to supplement and medication interactions, and I cannot prescribe supplements and/or medication. If you are unclear about a supplement, how to use it, or how it may affect your body, please ask your doctor.

Cravings

Before we dive into your 21 days, I must address cravings.

Right now, you likely have them, and they have probably gone wild. You might start eating a few chips or a single cookie, but then end up eating the entire bag or box. Your gut bacteria are *craving* for you to continue feeding it, which results in more rotten gut bacteria, leaving you feeling famished and possibly encouraging extra pounds to linger.

During these 21 days you will, without a doubt, have a craving here or there (or maybe even for several days at a time). This is normal, but you must understand that to overcome them, you must stop them in their tracks.

Some tips to help you control cravings:

1. **Stay hydrated.** Don't let your body get too thirsty. We often experience dehydration as mild hunger. Try drinking a glass of water first thing when you wake up in the morning, after you've been "fasting" all night long, to jump-start your day with proper hydration. Bonus: a great morning bowel movement.

2. **Fill your craving with something other than food.** Oftentimes, eating becomes a substitute for entertainment, or a way to fill in a void in our lives. However, ask yourself what you're *really* feeling. If it's boredom, loneliness, or another emotion, address those feelings with something other than food.

3. **Make sure you're getting enough nutrients.** Following the Gutsy Girl's 21-day plan should *not* mean you cannot get adequate nutrients. Make sure to drink broths, eat real foods,

continued on page 86

UNDERSTANDING LOW STOMACH ACID

Low stomach acid, also called hypochlorhydria, is a condition where the body doesn't produce enough acid to break down proteins into the essential amino acids and nutrients the body needs.

Despite what the drug industry may tell us, stomach acid is not a bad thing. In fact, stomach acid is needed in order to break food down. In a well-functioning system, hydrochloric acid (HCL) converts or activates pepsinogen to pepsin, which digests proteins. The amount of HCL in the body decreases as we age. Oftentimes when people go to their doctors and tell them they are experiencing acid reflux, they will be given an antacid and sent on their way.[1] But the antacid, of course, only reduces stomach acid even more, masking the problem and causing a harsh ripple effect.

Low stomach acid can be responsible for a whole host of symptoms, including diarrhea, gas, bloating, acid reflux, excessive burping, heartburn, nausea after eating, undigested food in stools, headaches, difficulty digesting meat, weight gain, acne, eczema, hair loss, brittle nails, allergies, iron deficiency, vitamin B_{12} deficiency, and even malnutrition, because your body isn't absorbing essential nutrients. If left untreated, other related signs can include reduced liver function, ulcers, chronic intestinal infections, hypothyroidism, low white blood cell count, chronic fatigue, adrenal fatigue, and an increased risk of gallstones. And low stomach acid is often associated with disorders including SIBO, IBS, IBS, leaky gut syndrome, diabetes, candida, and autoimmune diseases in general.

THE HCL CHALLENGE TEST

If you suspect you may have low stomach acid, there are a few different ways you can test for it at home. The betaine HCL challenge is the one

---

[1] http://chriskresser.com/how-your-antacid-drug-is-making-you-sick-part-b/

that has been most effective for me. Always consult your health practitioner before conducting an HCL challenge test on your own. Note: This is especially important if you take NSAIDs or corticosteroids, as taking them together with HCL can increase your risk of gastritis.

To complete the HCL challenge test at home, all you'll need is betaine HCL (preferably with pepsin) and a protein-heavy meal. To conduct the test:

1. Prepare a meal containing at least 4 to 6 ounces of protein.
2. Begin eating the meal. Halfway through, stop and take one betaine HCL pill and then finish your meal.
3. Listen to your body.

Does your stomach feel perfectly normal, or do you feel a burning sensation?

If, after doing the challenge with just one betaine HCL pill, you feel a burning sensation, you likely have enough stomach acid. If not, try the challenge again, but this time take two betaine HCL pills instead of one. Continue trying the challenge until you feel the burning sensation (but do not increase to more than six pills), and make note of how many pills it takes to cause a reaction. The more you have to take, the more likely it is that you do not have enough stomach acid. If you reach six or more betaine HCL pills with no effects, please contact your doctor before increasing even more. They will likely have a different approach they may want you to try.

If you do find that you have low stomach acid, betaine HCL can be used alongside natural dietary methods to help your body naturally begin producing more HCL. When I first did the HCL challenge test, I was able to take twelve—yes, twelve—pills with *zero* burning sensations. Over time, I was able to gradually reduce the number of HCL pills

I needed to four per high-protein meal, and today I only take them sporadically in a smaller dose when needed.

HOW TO NATURALLY IMPROVE STOMACH ACID PRODUCTION

While betaine HCL can help kick-start your body's HCL production, you can also help to naturally increase it with dietary changes. Here are a few of the best ways to improve stomach acid production without supplements:

1. Add fermented veggies to your diet. You can make your own fermented veggies or buy sauerkraut, kimchi, and other fermented products from brands like Bubbies and Farmhouse Culture. If you can't handle the full product, try just the juice, which also helps.
2. Use a quality sea salt. Pink Himalayan salt is my favorite because not only can it help with acid production, it also contains important minerals like magnesium, which helps reduce stress levels and is great for those recovering from adrenal fatigue.
3. Explore food combining. Carbohydrates reduce the production of HCL, while protein requires HCL to be digested, so if you can avoid mixing the two, it can help. (That said, it's more important to cut down on stress, so if this one will stress you out, skip it.)
4. Marinate your meats. You can marinate meat prior to cooking with lemon, lime, or apple cider vinegar to help your body more easily digest the protein.
5. Chew. Take your time when eating meals. Did you know that digestion begins in the mouth, and that you have digestive enzymes there as well? Chew your food slowly to

break it down as much as possible before it even reaches the stomach.

6. Drink hot liquids rather than cold at mealtimes. Ice water inhibits the production of stomach acid, so avoid drinking it with your meals.

7. Choose your beverages wisely. Ginger, dandelion root, and lemon all naturally increase HCL production. You can make your own warm infused beverage, or easier yet, try caffeine-free Ginger Aid® or roasted dandelion root teas.

8. Stay calm. Overall stomach acid levels drop as we become more stressed. Learn to manage your stress, especially around mealtimes, so that your body can focus on its job and digest food.

9. Eliminate all food sensitivities. If you're following the 21-day plan, you're probably already doing this, but it's important to note that consuming foods you are sensitive or intolerant to on a daily basis causes a decrease in stomach acid production.

10. Add apple cider vinegar to your diet wherever you can. You can mix a little in with water and drink it before each meal, or better yet, cook with it. Bragg Organic Raw Apple Cider Vinegar® is my favorite.

and pay attention to the variety in your diet to ensure proper nutrition and reduce your cravings.

4. **Pay attention to your hormones.** When women experience menstruation, pregnancy, or menopause, fluctuating estrogen levels may cause unusual cravings. While this is common, it's not (necessarily) normal. However, when this happens, figure out exactly what it is you're craving and then identify an appropriate substitute for it. Want pizza? Instead of calling the local delivery boy, make your own from ingredients on the "Say Yes" list. Or maybe you want ice cream? Instead of grabbing the carton in your freezer, try making "nice-cream" by blending a frozen banana and the nondairy milk of your choice.

Remember, cravings are not the enemy. It's how you act upon your cravings that will determine how quickly you progress (or regress) in healing your gut.

LIFESTYLE

Diagnosis and diet can go a long way toward repairing your gut and rebuilding your health. But you may find that even after you have an appropriate diagnosis and have figured out the diet that's right for you, some of your symptoms persist. The last piece of the healing puzzle, and by far the most difficult one to conquer, is changing your lifestyle.

If you want the honest, real, and raw truth, it's within the lifestyle pillar that most of your healing will or will not occur. The lifestyle pillar includes movement (exercise, workouts, whatever you want to call it), stress reduction, sleep, skin and body care, and many other critical factors that can affect your health. It may or may not also include supplements and/or medications.

Lifestyle changes are the part of the equation that everyone knows they need, even if they don't want to admit it.

And though we're starting here with just 21 days, making these changes will, without a doubt, be a lifelong journey.

Get Moving

When healing the gut, I believe that walking is, by far, the best form of movement and exercise. While I do not believe that intense exercise and gut healing can coexist, it's also true that *no* exercise and gut healing cannot coexist. In my own journey, I found that I needed to keep my body moving to heal, but every time I tried to tell myself, "Okay, I'm all better. Time to work out hard again" before I truly *was* better, a relapse showed up.

Finding the right balance is hard for many women, especially when we've been programmed to run like a hamster on a wheel for years.

The solution? Just walk. I cannot emphasize enough how incredibly healing a simple daily walk can be. When I healed my gut for the last time, walking was pretty much the one and only form of exercise I did for almost a year. Walking is powerful on many levels. It keeps everything moving, keeps the lymphatic system circulating, and is a form of cardio without the stress many other forms put on the body.

Even if you walk slowly, you're still moving forward. And such is the healing journey.

Sleep and Gut Healing

The connection between sleep and gut healing is so important. (In fact, if you're up late reading this and sacrificing sleep time, stop now, close this book, and go to bed!) When I began journaling and using a device to track my sleep, I immediately noticed a critical pattern. On days where I'd gotten less than 8 hours of sleep the night before, I would feel fatigued, unable to work out, and would be starving throughout the day.

When I got more than 8 hours of sleep, though, my journal entries would say things like "Lovely day" and "I felt amazing." I had the energy to work out and was much less hungry; I was able to eat an adequate amount of food and feel satisfied.

The National Sleep Foundation says that adults (26 to 64 years old) need 7 to 9 hours of sleep per night.[15] And while I believe this is a great guideline, the ideal number of hours for you will depend on your own unique situation and your other lifestyle factors. For me, I've found that anything less than 8 hours leaves me nearly empty. Truth be told, I have even noticed a difference between how I feel on 7 hours and 45 minutes of sleep versus 8 hours and 15 minutes. That extra 30 minutes changes my whole day.

Sleep, or a lack thereof, can have a huge effect on full gut healing. In "8 Scary Signs of Sleep Deprivation," the *Huffington Post* reports a few of the signs that you may not be getting enough sleep: "you're ravenous, you're weepy and you can't shake that cold."[16]

Getting enough sleep is imperative for your healing efforts. Here are some ways to ensure that you're getting the right amount of sleep for you:

1. Remember, your house does not have to be perfectly clean. Sleep is more important, so make it a priority.
2. Stop being a night owl. Netflix will still be there tomorrow.
3. Place an aromatherapy diffuser next to your bed to help you relax.
4. Get blue-light glasses to help you block blue light (from phones, computer screens, etc.) closer to bedtime, so the blue light doesn't disrupt your sleep.
5. Create a sleep-friendly environment. This looks different for everyone, but think about your ideal sleep temperature, light level, noise level, and scents and adjust your bedroom to optimize your sleeping environment.

Sleep like your healing journey depends on it. To a degree, it does.

---

[15] https://www.sleepfoundation.org/how-sleep-works/how-much-sleep-do-we-really-need
[16] https://www.huffpost.com/entry/scary-sleep-deprivation-effects_n_2807026

Endocrine Disruptors: Skin and Body Care

I had a nose rash that plagued me off and on for years, starting when I was just 13 years old. After countless misdiagnoses, I finally learned what it really was: perioral dermatitis (PD). According to the American Osteopathic College of Dermatology (AOCD):

> Perioral dermatitis is a facial rash that tends to occur around the mouth. Most often it is red and slightly scaly or bumpy. Any itching or burning is mild. It may spread up around the nose, and occasionally the eyes while avoiding the skin adjacent to the lips. It is more rare in men and children. Perioral dermatitis may come and go for months or years.[17]

What, you may be wondering, does all this have to do with gut health? Well, if you dig deep, you'll find that the root cause of PD is often, you guessed it, *the gut*. It's associated with an overgrowth of gut bacteria of sorts.

Skin health and gut health, it turns out, are often closely related. The foundation for good skin health starts from within. If your insides aren't well, nothing you use topically—no face wash, moisturizer, or makeup—will make a difference in your skin's appearance. That said, if what you're using topically isn't as high quality as the food you're using to nourish your body, you must know that damage is being done. It's important to remember that problems such as these are not *only* caused by food—there are so many external factors that can contribute as well. In my case, my doctor determined my diet was likely not the culprit.

There are many theories around what causes perioral dermatitis and/or triggers it to come back, and I found that the key to healing my own rash was to search my topical body care products for endocrine disruptors. Endocrine disruptors are chemicals that may interfere with the body's

---

[17]https://www.aocd.org/page/PerioralDermatitis

continued on page 92

DO YOU HAVE ROTTEN GUT BACTERIA?

A craving for sweet and starchy foods is typical for all people with abnormal bodily flora, particularly with Candida albicans *overgrowth. No matter how finicky, most would accept sugary drinks, biscuits, cakes, sweets, sugar-laden breakfast cereals, chocolates, chips, crisps, pasta and white bread. In fact, these are the foods to which many people limit their diet thus feeding the vicious circle of abnormal flora and toxicity in their bodies.*[1]

When I was in college and in my early twenties, I ate a lot of fat-free, sugar-free junk. And I ate a *ton* on a day-to-day basis, because I was starving all the time. I also produced quite a stench, which is how I know I had a rotten gut. You can probably tell if you, too, have rotten gut bacteria. This is becoming a more and more common issue because of the food we eat and the lifestyles we live. And because many people don't want to admit to their rotten gut bacteria, they just keep on living the same way, while their rotten gut bacteria multiplies rapidly.

Growing evidence suggests that "bad bacteria boost appetite, which may explain why some people struggle more with weight gain than others."[2] When the gut is filled with rotten bacteria, it craves more rotten foods to keep the rotten bacteria satisfied, and often prohibits the absorption of necessary nutrients. This causes us to become even hungrier, with even more cravings, and the cycle continues. Unwanted weight gain is often the result, since we tend to gain weight when junk

---

[1]*Gut and Psychology Syndrome: Natural Treatment for Autism, Dyspraxia, A.D.D., Dyslexia, A.D.H.D., Depression, Schizophrenia*, by Dr. Natasha Campbell-McBride
[2]http://www.dailymail.co.uk/health/article-1258221/Overweight-Blame-bad-gut-bacteria-boost-appetite.html

calories are consumed instead of quality calories.[3] With rotten gut bacteria and a hungry appetite, we are up against a never-ending battle.

If this all sounds familiar, you must begin to eat real food, but you also must understand that there is far more to it than just "real food." If you have severe IBS and/or IBD, simply avoiding junk food and junk ingredients is probably not enough. Until your gut has healed, even much of your "real food" is probably keeping you symptomatic (and smelly). You may need a special diet protocol to "starve" your gut bacteria for a while and help reset your body. There are five primary diet protocols that help starve gut bacteria: paleo (maybe even AIP), the GAPS diet, SCD, low-FODMAP, and occasionally, the elemental diet. For more on these diet protocols and how they can help, see page 49.

---

[3]http://health.usnews.com/health-news/blogs/eat-run/2013/07/08/consider-the-quality-and-quantity-of-calories

endocrine system and produce adverse developmental, reproductive, neurological, and immune effects in both humans and wildlife.[18]

Unfortunately, these chemicals are often found in topical skin and body care products, and they can have dramatic effects on your body. According to the Environmental Working Group (EWG):

> There is no end to the tricks that endocrine disruptors can play on our bodies: increasing production of certain hormones; decreasing production of others; imitating hormones; turning one hormone into another; interfering with hormone signaling; telling cells to die prematurely; competing with essential nutrients; binding to essential hormones; accumulating in organs that produce hormones.[19]

The EWG has published a list of what they call the "Dirty Dozen Endocrine Disruptors":[20]

1. BPA
2. Dioxin
3. Atrazine
4. Phthalates
5. Perchlorate
6. Fire retardants
7. Lead
8. Arsenic
9. Mercury
10. Perfluorinated chemicals (PFCs)
11. Organophosphate pesticides
12. Glycol ethers

---

[18]https://www.niehs.nih.gov/health/topics/agents/endocrine/index.cfm
[19]https://www.ewg.org/consumer-guides/dirty-dozen-endocrine-disruptors#.WghFLRNSzBJ
[20]https://www.ewg.org/consumer-guides/dirty-dozen-endocrine-disruptors#.Wj0AxVQ-fq2

When I started looking into these, I realized that I'd been using products with those 12 things in them for years. I now watch for the Dirty Dozen in anything and everything I buy, and it's made a big difference in my skin and gut health. I encourage you to do the same.

The Never List

The more I dug into what was really in all those skin and body care products, the more I realized just how many ingredients were doing more harm than good.

We spend so much time analyzing and overanalyzing every thing we put into our bodies, but so many of us never think twice about the things we put on our skin. If you're doing the hard work of making dietary changes and following the "Say Yes" and "Say No" lists on pages 54–55 and 62–72, carry that idea through to the other parts of your lifestyle as well and pay attention to the ingredients in your skincare products. I've compiled the following list of "Never" ingredients to stay away from for optimal skin and gut health (see pages 94–95).

Now, if you use one of these ingredients every now and then, will you die? Of course not. But the more we know, the better our decisions can be. Get into the habit of searching product labels for these ingredients and see Resources (page 252) for my favorite safe cosmetic and skin care brands.

It's also true that sometimes the healing measures we take for our insides can have a temporary negative effect on our skin. For a couple of weeks at the start of my healing process, for example, I had to "starve" my gut bacteria with a low-FODMAP diet. Because high-FODMAP honey was off-limits during this time, I ended up consuming more stevia than usual. I was using pure, organic liquid stevia, so I didn't expect any issues, but when someone mentioned to me that stevia caused her cystic acne to flare, a lightbulb went on in my head. Could the stevia I was using as part of my gut-repair diet be causing the cystic back acne I'd been dealing with? Sure enough, when I cut out the stevia, my back began to heal almost immediately.

continued on page 96

"NEVER" LIST

Benzalkonium chloride	A chemical disinfectant that's used in everything from cleaning products to sunscreens and laundry materials to moisturizers. Potential side effects include irritation to the eyes, skin, and respiratory system.[1]
BHA and BHT	Both BHA (butylhydroxyanisole) and BHT (butylhydroxytoluene) are commonly used as synthetic preservatives to extend shelf life. Both food and cosmetic manufacturers use them for everything from packaged foods to lipsticks, diaper creams, and deodorants. Potential side effects include irritation to the skin and organ damage (including the possibility of liver damage).[2]
Ethanolamine (MEA/DEA/TEA)	Used as emulsifiers and pH adjustors, you'll find these in things like fragrances, cleaning supplies, and cosmetics. Potential side effects include toxicity to the skin and organs, including male reproductive health and general hormone disruption.[3]
Formaldehyde	Formaldehyde is flammable and toxic preservative that's commonly found in building materials, but also prevalent in the cosmetics industry via lotion, makeup, and shampoo. Potential side effects include neurotoxicity, and even cancer.[4]
Hydroquinone	A cream that makes the skin lighter, it's mostly found in products intended to lighten the skin (i.e., skin brightening creams). Potential side effects include skin irritation (including a stinging sensation), inflammation and overall irritation.[5]
Methyl-isothiazolinone and methyl-chloroisothiazolinone	Common chemical preservatives used in cleaning products, sunscreen, personal care products (namely shampoo and conditioner), and other cosmetics. Potential side effects include dermatitis and other skin sensitivities and allergies.[6]
Parabens (methyl-, isobutyl-, propyl- and others)	Preservatives that are used to prevent mold and bacterial overgrowth. They are found in cosmetics, shampoo, conditioner, lotion, and body wash. Potential side effects include hormone disruption, reduced sperm production, and potentially cancer.[7]
Phthalates (DBP, DEHP, DEP and others)	Though they are banned in the European Union, these plasticizing chemicals are still commonly used in the United States. You'll find them in nail polish, fragrances, hair care products, and other plastics. Potential side effects include endocrine system disruption and reproductive toxicity.[8]
Polyethylene glycol (PEG compounds)	I've discussed this ingredient many times as it relates to MiraLax (for treating constipation), but PEG is the main ingredient in anti-freeze. It's used as a thickener, penetration enhancement (ease of ingredients entering the body), and even as a softener. You will find it in everything from creams and sunscreen to household cleaners and laxatives. Potential side effects include links to cancer (via ethylene oxide through the ethoxylation process).[9]

"NEVER" LIST

Retinyl palmitate and retinol (Vitamin A)	Vitamin A? What's wrong with Vitamin A? This is an ingredient that is used to slow the aging process. However, retinyl palmitate, which is a form of vitamin A, has been shown to speed skin tumor growth and cause things like brittle nails and hair loss when used topically. You find it in antiaging products, namely, moisturizers.[10]
Sodium lauryl sulfate and sodium laureth sulfate (SLS and SLES)	Produce the bubbles and foam various products make when lathered. It's found in products like shampoo, face wash, bubble bath, and body wash. Potential side effects include skin and eye irritation and triggered allergies.[11]
Synthetic flavor or fragrance	Chemical combinations used to create a flavor or fragrance (sometimes up to 3,000 different chemicals are used in a single synthetic compound). Manufacturers are not required to disclose what is in any fragranced formula. These are found in all types of foods, cosmetics, household cleaning products, personal care products–everything! Potential side effects include disruption of hormones, allergies, and other health problems.[12]
Toluene	A clear liquid that has a distinct smell. It is mostly found in nail polish and paint thinner. Potential side effects include birth defects, immune system problems, and neurological complications.[13]
Triclosan and triclocarban	Used as antimicrobials, you'll find these ingredients most in hand sanitizers and other cleansing agents like soap and even toothpaste). In addition to being endocrine disruptors and having impacts on human reproduction, another massive issue is they are toxic to the environment (namely aquatics).[14]

[1] https://www.ncbi.nlm.nih.gov/pmc/articles/PMC6581159/
[2] https://www.madesafe.org/chemical-profiles/bht-and-bha/
[3] https://www.safecosmetics.org/get-the-facts/chemicals-of-concern/ ethanolamine-compounds/
[4] https://www.cancer.org/cancer/cancer-causes/formaldehyde.html
[5] https://www.ncbi.nlm.nih.gov/books/NBK539693/
[6] https://www.ncbi.nlm.nih.gov/pmc/articles/PMC4056723/
[7] https://www.safecosmetics.org/get-the-facts/chemicals-of-concern/parabens/
[8] https://www.safecosmetics.org/get-the-facts/chemicals-of-concern/phthalates/
[9] https://www.madesafe.org/chemicalcallout-polyethylene-glycol-compounds-pegs/
[10] https://www.ewg.org/sunscreen/the-problem-with-vitamin-a/
[11] https://davidsuzuki.org/queen-of-green/dirty-dozen-sodium-laureth-sulfate/
[12] https://www.ewg.org/foodscores/content/natural-vs-artificial-flavors/
[13] https://pubchem.ncbi.nlm.nih.gov/compound/Toluene
[14] https://www.ncbi.nlm.nih.gov/pmc/articles/PMC5644973/

Skincare companies would like you to believe that their products are necessary for skin healing, but my motto is, *Minimizing is maximizing.* To heal my cystic acne, I didn't have to add any products at all. I simply had to remove what wasn't working and focus on the root of the problem, not the symptom itself.

WHEN THE JEANS DON'T FIT

As women, we are told that when the jeans don't fit, the solution is to go on a diet and lose weight. I, too, believed this for almost my whole life. But once my gut began to heal, I realized that the solution is actually much simpler: Just buy yourself some jeans that fit.

Once when I was vacationing in Lake Tahoe, it had been almost a year since I'd last worn my outdoor ski pants and jacket. When I put them on, I was shocked to find that *both* pieces were tight all around. I won't lie—for the first several minutes, I thought, "Definitely need to cut back and lose a few pounds!" But those thoughts didn't last long. I remembered that back when these ski pants and jacket had fit much better, I felt awful most of the time and often had to unbutton my pants due to bloating. My weight might have been lower on the scale, but I was definitely not happy, no matter what it looked like on the outside. Now, though, with a healthy gut, I've found so much peace in the ability to *just eat,* to exercise for pleasure, and to enjoy food with family and friends at any given moment. This has allowed me to *naturally* crave less junk, to eat when I'm hungry, and to get off the daily roller-coaster ride of up-and-down weight and emotions. My digestive systems functions the way it should, and I am at a place that my body has been desperately trying to get to for a very long time. From this place, I was able to see that the solution was not a new diet. The solution was simple: I just needed bigger ski pants and a new jacket.

ONE CHANGE FOR PERIORAL DERMATITIS

Back in 2014, I wrote a blog post explaining how I had healed my perioral dermatitis with the GAPS diet, more consistent sleep, and a variety of dietary supplements and other lifestyle changes. One of the specific changes I noted was that I had stopped using all traditional toothpaste, which usually contains sodium lauryl sulfate and fluoride. A few years later, when I started seeing the perioral dermatitis around my nose again, I immediately thought, "It must be the diet." But adjusting my diet didn't help, and over a month later, I couldn't figure out why my rash hadn't improved. Then one day, while I was brushing my teeth with the "all natural, fluoride-free" Tom's of Maine toothpaste I'd grabbed at Target, I took a closer look at the ingredients:

Calcium carbonate, glycerin, water, xylitol, hydrated silica, natural flavor (peppermint oil), sodium lauryl sulfate, zinc citrate, carra-geenan, sodium bicarbonate

I don't know why I had assumed that Tom's of Maine didn't use SLS (maybe because it said fluoride-free, I thought I was in the clear?), but there it was, clearly written on the label: sodium lauryl sulfate.

I immediately switched to the Earthpaste-brand toothpaste that contained only five ingredients and no SLS or other foaming agents, and two days later, my nose was 100% healed.

Turns out it wasn't my diet after all, and the incident reminded me yet again that food is not always the enemy. If you have lingering perioral dermatitis issues, check your toothpaste. This one change could be the key for you, too.

And don't just think SLS is in your toothpaste—it's everywhere.

THOUGHTS ON ANTIBIOTICS

I've always preached a doctrine of healing with food and lifestyle, not drugs and medication.

Living unprocessed is the only way for me. I eat healthy, I prioritize clean living, I love my essential oils, and I always avoid drugs and antibiotics whenever possible. But all of that is *prevention*, not *intervention*. I live my life based on prevention, and I do a good job at it, which means I rarely need antibiotics. Yet there are times and places when intervention is absolutely needed, and the truth is, antibiotics can be lifesaving. If you find yourself in a place where you truly need to take an antibiotic to preserve your health, do it, and don't feel shame.

According to the National Library of Medicine, antibiotics are "powerful medicines that fight bacterial infections. Used properly, antibiotics can save lives. They either kill bacteria or keep them from reproducing. Your body's natural defenses can usually take it from there."[1]

The problem with antibiotics, though, is that as a society, we have used them too much and too often, and "the overuse of antibiotics clearly drives the evolution of resistance." Antibiotics work for bacterial, not viral, infections, so when people take them for viruses like colds, flu, and most coughs, sore throats, and bouts of bronchitis, they can actually do more harm than good, enabling bacteria to change and become more resistant to the antibiotic.

Antibiotics can also cause major side effects, including stomach problems like diarrhea, nausea, and vomiting; thrush infections; allergic reactions such as hives, fever, and breathing problems; menstrual cycle problems; tendon ruptures; and hallucinations or psychotic reactions, and more.[2]

---

[1] https://medlineplus.gov/antibiotics.html
[2] https://draxe.com/health/antibiotic-side-effects/

If you're already experiencing gut-health issues, obviously the digestive side effects will be of particular concern. Fortunately, there are a number of simple and practical ways you can rebuild your gut after antibiotics:

1. Take a probiotic. I highly recommend the Just Thrive brand.
2. Eat prebiotics freely, but responsibly. (You can even ferment your own food at home.)
3. Give your system a break. Consider intermittent fasting and meal spacing for a few weeks.
4. Reduce or eliminate sugar in your diet. Sugar loves to feed bacteria.
5. Rebuild the gut lining with foods and supplements like bone broth, collagen, and L-glutamine.
6. If you can tolerate them, eat a lot of veggies, greens, and fiber. They will help add bulk to the stool to flush the antibiotics through your system.
7. Know your own triggers, and remove any and all foods that might be causing you digestive distress.
8. Sleep. Seriously. It's as great for healing the gut as it is for healing your life.

An ounce of prevention is worth a pound of cure, so you should absolutely do everything you can to avoid having to take antibiotics in the first place. But when you do need them, take them and get better, so you can get back to healing your gut.

A GUTSY GIRL'S
21-DAY PLAN

Welcome to your 21-day journey to a healthier, calmer, happier you. The 21-day plan is a *temporary* elimination diet. It is meant to reset your body so that you can start rebuilding your gut health and finding the diet and lifestyle plan that is 100% customized to and for you, for life.

As you progress through the 21 days, don't forget to keep track of your progress and record your thoughts and feelings in your journal each day. You can use the space in the margins of this book for these purposes, or grab any journal or notebook that inspires you. At agutsygirl.com I also offer a 90-day gut-healing journal, *Healing Blooms from Within*, which you can use throughout this 21-day plan and beyond.

This is not like every other 21-, 30-, or 60-day elimination diet or gut-healing plan. In fact, I don't know of any other plan for gut healing (or gut health) like this one on the market. When I was on my own healing journey, I read books upon books upon books. My favorite health and healing books were the minimal ones, because I could take the information someone else had provided, meditate on it, and then mark the book up with how and why it related to my own experiences, my own journey.

By the time I was done with a book, not only was I more knowledge-able, but the book was also filled with various colors of ink and Post-its. I could then go back at any given moment and know exactly what was mine, because it was all right there in color and texture.

I've tried to mirror this with the book you're holding in your hands and the 21-day journey you're about to go on. Through these next 21 days, I will share my own stories and advice. The structure of my plan is all right there in black and white, and there is space in the margin to accompany the bland black and white. This was very intentional. My hope is that you'll add your own color by journaling your thoughts and putting these suggestions into action in your own life.

So, what does each day of the 21-day plan include? Every day, I'll share a story with you from my own journey to help you understand more about why this is all so important, and hopefully inspire you to make your own changes. Each day also includes a list of daily actions that are critical to take, bonus actions you can take if you're feeling up to it, recipe "Creation" ideas to help you get on the right track with your diet, and a "Gut Real" thought or tip for the day.

You'll notice that the daily list of critical actions is the same each day, and it appears *every single day*. This is because these actions are so impor-tant, you need to do them every single day throughout the course of this journey.

Your Daily Critical Actions Include:

- ☐ Getting at least 8 hours of sleep
- ☐ Recording all bowel movements (time and type)
- ☐ Following the "Say Yes" and "Say No" lists on pages 54–55 and 62–72, choosing meals from the Gutsy Girl's Creations chapter on page 212, and recording what you're eating. Be sure to record *all* the ingredients—not just the "ingredient(s)" (see below).
- ☐ Consuming at least 8 cups of water
- ☐ Writing one line of gratitude and/or your daily mantra

- [ ] Choosing a workout activity that ranks no more than a 5 on an intensity scale of 1 to 10, and working out for a *brief* period of time
- [ ] Doing one thing that your practitioner has told you to do, but you have not done yet. This is something your doctor, nutritionist, or other medical provider has advised that you know you should do, but have been putting off—you may have one thing in mind, or a few, depending on your situation. (For me, this was taking HCL with my high-protein meals every single day.)
- [ ] Recording what cycle day (CD) you're on for your menstrual cycle (CD 1 = the day your period starts), if applicable.

NOTE: If you've chosen to use my *Healing Blooms from Within* journal to record your thoughts, most of the above (and much more!) is already pre-populated for you on each page.

ONE FINAL NOTE BEFORE YOU BEGIN: If you have a family to feed, don't think you have to make one meal for them and one for you throughout these 21 days. My family ate the same meal as me each night for dinner. The *only* difference was that they might add a specific food item I chose not to have. Keep it practical, make it simple, and work together as a family to discover how you can heal.

INGREDIENTS VS. INGREDIENT(S)

Keeping track of what you're eating sounds simple enough, but it's important to realize there are ingredients, and then there are what I like to call "ingredient(s)." True ingredients are whole, pure, untouched foods that can be combined to create a new food. Whole fruits and vegetables, raw nuts, rice, herbs, and unprocessed fish and meats are all ingredients. Ingredient(s), however, are individual food items that are actually made up of many different ingredients. A premade salad dressing or cake mix, for example, may be listed as a single "ingredient" in a recipe. But if you look at the label, you'll see that the single bottle or box actually contains many individual ingredients.

Why is this important for the Gutsy Girl? If you are trying to heal your gut, you need to be hyperaware of the difference between ingredients and ingredient(s) as you embark on your 21-day elimination diet. You also need to keep it in mind as you're journaling your daily food intake. Early in on my journey, while working hard to understand which foods my body was reacting to, I would record everything I ate in a day. A sample list might include, for example, brown rice, salmon, olive oil, and Simple Mills Chocolate Muffin Mix. Everything was healthy, gluten-free, paleo, and dairy-free, so I couldn't understand why I was having a reaction. But when I dug deeper and read the small print on the muffin mix, I realized it actually contained ingredients that were *not* low-FODMAP. Committing to your gut-healing journey means you need to pay attention to every single ingredient you eat, including those that are hidden within prepared and packaged "ingredient(s)." Of course, recording these detailed ingredient lists can get overwhelming, and that's why I urge you to eat whole foods in their natural state, and stay away from processed and packaged foods, as much as possible during this 21-day journey.

NOTES

It was 2012, and I was hiking down the Grand Canyon in Arizona when these five words hit me like a 500-pound sack of bricks: *nothing changes if nothing changes.*

It had been a long year of struggling with my health, trying various drugs, steroids, and antibiotics, barely moving my body and going, going, going for up to 10 hours a day without focusing enough on the food and supplements that were critical for me. I was going through various infertility treatments, which culminated in an IVF (in vitro fertilization) cycle. As I traveled near Sedona that April, I was looking back and reflecting, writing out my frustrations, how I had been feeling, what was working, and what was not working.

In the end, I realized more things were not working than were working. And with those five words echoing in my mind—nothing changes if nothing changes—I knew it was time to start on a new path.

Old habits die hard, and though I began making many changes in that season of my life, it took a long time for me to ultimately find my way. And along the journey, I had to learn and relearn the meaning of these five words.

Change is hard, especially when it seems to disrupt the only way we know how to live. But when "the only way we know how to live" is killing us physically or emotionally, those hard changes are necessary. It takes a strong woman to make real change, to *really* look within and decide that excuses can no longer be a part of her equation.

NOTES

You are doing hard things today, as you were yesterday. And if you're being honest with yourself you also know that change, no matter how small or large, must happen.

Today marks the beginning of your own journey on the true path to healing. One simple change might be all you need to start today.

I have poured my heart and soul into giving you the material you need to succeed, along with the confidence to make it happen. What stands between how you feel today and the gut healing that will begin to happen over these next few weeks (and for the rest of your life) is *you*.

Ultimately, you are the only one who can make change happen.

Beginnings bring fear, and that's okay. In his book *Resilience*, Eric Greitens writes that the fear that comes with beginnings is good: "It tells you that you are on the cusp of something worthwhile."[1] And I really think you are onto the most worthwhile thing you might have ever done for yourself. You are not wishing anymore; you are doing.

Take deep breaths, enjoy your food, and *embrace the process*. It's your time to move forward, make big changes, and have your gut feeling like it never has before.

This 21-day plan is super simple, but your 21 days will not be easy. Remember, though, it's just 21 days, and most of the things in life that are not easy are worth it in the end. I hated the beginning

---

[1]*Resilience: Hard-Won Wisdom for Living a Better Life,* Eric Greitens

of my own first 21-day journey. I love where I am today. And I know that once you begin down this road of change, you'll love where you end up, too.

CRITICAL ACTIONS TO TAKE TODAY:

☐ Get at least 8 hours of sleep.

☐ Record all bowel movements (time and type).

☐ Follow the "Say Yes" and "Say No" lists on pages 54–55 and 62–72.

☐ Choose meals from the Creations chapter on page 212.

☐ Record what you're eating—*all* the ingredients, not just the "ingredient(s)" (see page 103).

☐ Consume at least 8 cups of water.

☐ Write one line of gratitude and/or your healing mantra.

☐ Choose a workout activity that ranks no more than a 5 on an intensity scale of 1 to 10, and work out for a brief period of time.

☐ Do one thing your practitioner has told you to do but you just have not done yet.

☐ Record what cycle day (CD) you're on for your menstrual cycle (CD 1 = the day your period starts).

ACTIONS TO CONSIDER TAKING TODAY:

☐ **Begin your own journal.** Even if you are keeping an electronic food journal, I highly recommend a handwritten one as well. I often return to the first handwritten journal I ever kept on my own journey, and I am always frustrated that I only wrote through Day 11, since it was on Day 20 that my life truly began to change. Write down anything of note. You might be surprised at what you find out about yourself, your health, and your general well-being while exploring.

☐ **Take a picture.** Some people like to take a picture prior to change. I did back in April 2012. After months and months of drugs for IVF, I was bloated like none other. I was sick and miserable from drugs, antibiotics, and food. I love looking back on that misery as a simple reminder of where I've been, where I am now, and where I never want to be again.

☐ **Get on the scale.** Though the scale is not the best measurement of your well-being, you may want to weigh yourself today. As you heal, you might gain necessary weight you've been desperate to gain or you might lose weight due to decreased inflammation.

CREATION IDEAS FOR TODAY:

☐ Salmon Bowl (page 235)
☐ Beef, Chicken, or Vegetable Broth (page 240)
☐ Carrot Fries (page 248)

GUT REAL THOUGHT FOR TODAY:

Did you know that humans lack the digestive enzyme necessary to break down lactose? A small percentage of people will be able to tolerate dairy, but most cannot. Some have a very hard time digesting it even with the use of enzymes. You are likely one if you're reading this book. This is why we avoid dairy for these 21 days.

NOTES

If you've never hiked the Grand Canyon, it's a truly unique experience. Unlike most hikes I've been on, where you climb up and then get your "break" as you finish going back down, when you hike the Grand Canyon, you go down to climb back up.

On my way down the canyon, it all seemed so easy. The people traveling down with us were chatty, smiling, and feeling excited to be there. But as we passed those who were on the trek back up, I noticed a different tone; there was less talking, more sweating, solemn faces, and a lot of huffing and puffing.

I often realize so many things about life while I'm active, surrounded by nature, and left with nothing but the sound of my inner thoughts. During this hike, I thought a lot about the idea that what goes down must come up—and sometimes, coming up is the hardest part. You see, in life, we always think that when we're on a downward spiral, life is at its worst and is uncontrollable. Down equals the deepest and darkest; a difficult time.

But I'd argue that climbing back up is even more difficult. The real challenge in life is not how far you've fallen or the hurt and pain (physical and emotional) you've experienced in taking that fall. No, the real challenge is getting back up, climbing, and overcoming. Each step might bring blood, sweat, and tears, but without taking them you'll never get out of your internal Grand Canyon.

That day at the Grand Canyon, I didn't measure my success by the fact that I'd "fallen" 1,000+

feet—I measured it by how I climbed back up those same 1,000+ feet.

On this journey, you'll need to do the same.

SOUREST LEMON

Now let me give you a real-life example of how a time of physical and emotional pain led me to climb to reach a peak I didn't know existed.

Along with the rest of the world, I fell in love with the show *This Is Us* several years ago. In episode one of the show, the doctor says, "Take the sourest lemon life has to offer and turn it into something resembling lemonade." Well, my sourest lemon, at least up until now, has been infertility.

My husband and I spent years going through tests, trying every medical and nonmedical intervention possible. I allowed my body to be poked and prodded with nothing but hope and a positive attitude on my side. Throughout that time, I watched as friends quickly conceived, and for 12 to 16 days each cycle, I'd conjure up pregnancy symptoms in my mind and think, "I'm so pregnant this month."

I knew the 2-week wait signs and symptoms, and I was well acquainted with every last TTC (that's "trying to conceive") forum on the planet. I stalked them all, and every month what I read there had me convinced that surely I was pregnant.

But then, like clockwork, the stick would show one pink line.

Month after month, year after year, this continued, until the day my only successful IVF attempt ended in miscarriage. That day was one of the sourest in my life. In the days that followed, I felt an emptiness I can't describe. You will only understand if you've been in that place. I hope you have not.

But remember, this isn't a story about hiking down 1,000+ feet—it's a story about climbing back up. After the failed IVF, my husband and I took that trip to Sedona where we hiked the Grand Canyon. I believe it was a life-changing trip for both of us, individually and as a couple. We came back feeling renewed and ready to move forward. We didn't stand still wondering how to make another IVF cycle work, nor did we consider giving up altogether. Family is the most important thing in the world to us, and we knew we wanted it to consist of more than just the two of us and our dogs. So after the Sedona trip, we started climbing back out of the canyon. In just under 4 years, we went through the entire initial foster-to-adoption process and adopted our three beautiful babies: Samarah, Isaiah, and Amiya. After hitting the rock bottom of not being able to conceive naturally, we were able to turn around and head back out. The climb was not always easy; it was painful, both physically and emotionally, at times. But we saw it through, and with years of effort, we were able to reach the top.

Infertility was my sourest lemon. But today, I actually feel thankful for everything that has come to fruition because of it. No matter what your sourest lemon is, know that getting from sour to sweet will not always be an easy road. But someday you'll look back and say, "I can see it all so clearly now." You, too, can turn your sourest lemons into something resembling lemonade. In fact, something even better than lemonade. Maybe something more like kombucha or bone broth! As you continue on this path, don't allow your-self to feel discouraged or give up. Remember, you are leaps ahead of where most people are on their gut-healing journey. Why? Because you have taken the first step.

CRITICAL ACTIONS TO TAKE TODAY:

☐ Get at least 8 hours of sleep.

☐ Record all bowel movements (time and type).

☐ Follow the "Say Yes" and "Say No" lists on pages 54–55 and 62–72.

☐ Choose meals from the Creations chapter on page 212.

☐ Record what you're eating—*all* the ingredients, not just the "ingredient(s)" (see page 103).

☐ Consume at least 8 cups of water.

☐ Write one line of gratitude and/or your healing mantra.

☐ Choose a workout activity that ranks no more than a 5 on an intensity scale of 1 to 10, and work out for a brief period of time.

☐ Do one thing your practitioner has told you to do but you just have not done yet.

☐ Record what cycle day (CD) you're on for your

NOTES

menstrual cycle (CD 1 = the day your period starts).

ACTIONS FOR YOU TO CONSIDER TAKING TODAY:

☐ Journal. What is the "sourest lemon" in your own life?

☐ Take your own first step toward something, anything. Sure, you have already taken the first step with your gut health, but what's another first step you might be willing to take in another area of your life?

CREATION IDEAS FOR TODAY:

☐ Salad Bowl (page 234)

☐ Beef Bowl (page 237)

☐ Beef, Chicken, or Vegetable Broth (page 240)

GUT REAL THOUGHT FOR TODAY:

I know this is not easy. But I need to remind you that thinking of your 21 days like a diet will be the wrong approach. Remember, this is a temporary, 3-week transition. The point of it is to rid your body of all the things that continue to contribute to rotten feelings, and then move forward by adding things back in slowly to figure out what you are actually intolerant to, and what you can safely eat. (This, of course, is the best part!) You are far ahead of the game. You have taken the first step. You just need to continue on, because stopping only leads back to square one.

Perhaps you have heard the parable of the blind men and the elephant. To summarize, six blind men are touching an elephant. Each man is touching a different part of the elephant, so each man has a different answer to the question, "What are you touching?" Their answers range from "a wall" to "a type of snake."

All six men are touching a single, real object (the elephant), but because that object is so big, their viewpoints and experiences of what it might be are different. Each of the men only has one small piece of the puzzle. In order to identify what the elephant really is, they would need to connect all their individual experiences.

Healing your gut is like trying to identify that elephant with a blindfold on. As long as you're only approaching the issue from one angle, you will never find the complete answer. And each person who touches the act of gut healing will view and experience it in different ways. But there *is* one right answer—for the blind men, the answer is "elephant." And for you, the answer is "healed."

To arrive at that answer, you will need to draw on all your past experiences, make connections between what you're currently feeling and thinking, and ultimately spend enough time "moving about the elephant"—that is, looking at your gut health from every angle—to find the right approach.

When I first started my own healing journey, I was very much like the blind man only touching one small piece of the elephant. Knowing

NOTES

everything I know now, if I had to start my entire gut-healing journey over again, there are three things I would do right away, and I encourage you to do all three.

First, keep an extremely detailed food journal for at least 2 weeks, but ideally for all 21 days of this journey, or even a whole month. During this time, make no changes, and don't lie about anything you're eating or drinking or the way you're living. The more honest you are with yourself, the more accurate the next steps can be. And the more accurate the next steps are, the faster you will heal.

Once you've tracked your food and lifestyle patterns for a few weeks, review all the information and look for common themes. Where are you seeing patterns? Do certain foods cause symptoms? Is there something coming up with supplements and/or medications you're currently taking? Highlight the things that stand out most to you, and take your journal and your notes to your doctor to help guide their next steps.

Finally, begin to make changes based upon your results, and do only the things you need to do in order to heal. You might find you need a low-FODMAP diet, or you might not. You might need to go gluten-free, or maybe you'll be fine just switching to organic gluten. Or perhaps it was just a matter of low stomach acid all along.

If you've been spinning your wheels trying quick fixes with no results or using "Dr. Google" to drive your dietary and lifestyle changes, you're probably feeling frustrated, and that's because you're only looking at certain pieces of the puzzle; you're like the blind man who can only feel the elephant's leg. An honest and complete journal combined with the right diagnostic tests will allow you to begin to see the whole elephant for what it is.

CRITICAL ACTIONS TO TAKE TODAY:

- ☐ Get at least 8 hours of sleep.
- ☐ Record all bowel movements (time and type).
- ☐ Follow the "Say Yes" and "Say No" lists on pages 54–55 and 62–72.
- ☐ Choose meals from the Creations chapter on page 212.
- ☐ Record what you're eating—*all* the ingredients, not just the "ingredient(s)" (see page 103).
- ☐ Consume at least 8 cups of water.
- ☐ Write one line of gratitude and/or your healing mantra.
- ☐ Choose a workout activity that ranks no more than a 5 on an intensity scale of 1 to 10, and work out for a brief period of time.
- ☐ Do one thing your practitioner has told you to do but you just have not done yet.
- ☐ Record what cycle day (CD) you're on for your menstrual cycle (CD 1 = the day your period starts).

NOTES

ACTIONS FOR YOU TO CONSIDER TAKING TODAY:

☐ Journal. If you think about your gut health and healing journey as a whole, what is a piece of the puzzle you haven't yet focused on with full effort? What are three ways you can start focusing on that piece this week?

☐ Review your past food journal entries. Were you tracking total ingredients or just the main food label (e.g., ketchup)? If the latter, update those entries to add more detail. Are you seeing any patterns with what you are eating and how you are feeling?

CREATION IDEAS FOR TODAY:

☐ Springtime Protein Bowl (page 230)
☐ Beef, Chicken, or Vegetable Broth (page 240)
☐ Wild Alaskan Pollock (page 245)

GUT REAL THOUGHT FOR TODAY:

We always hear how important it is to be honest with other people. And while we also frequently hear, "Be honest with yourself," how often do we adhere to this advice? I'm telling you now—adhere to it. Get *really* honest with yourself for this journey. It's the only way you'll truly see yourself to the other side.

Half of this battle is mindset—in fact, it's probably a far greater percentage than half. Without the right mindset, it's nearly impossible to heal the gut.

So what is mindset, anyway? Your mindset is simply the established attitude you have toward something. *Psychology Today* says it is "a belief that orients the way we handle situations—the way we sort out what is going on and what we should do. Our mindsets help us spot opportunities, but they can also trap us in self-defeating cycles."[2]

Today, we're going to think about how your mindset relates to the way you feel about yourself, and how it relates to the way you view gut healing. The right mindset about both of these will set you up for success. You'll move with full conviction toward healing, and though success won't come overnight, it can and will happen. With a negative mindset, though, you'll be setting yourself up to fail. You've heard the saying and it's true: Whether you think you can or think you can't, you're right.

HOW YOU FEEL ABOUT YOURSELF

In order to find success in healing your gut, it's important to begin from a mindset of high self-esteem. When you look inward, if what you see and feel are negative, it makes it hard to heal. If

NOTES

---

[2] https://www.psychologytoday.com/us/blog/seeing-what-others-dont/201605/mindsets

you're constantly telling yourself you're not good enough, not worthy enough, and that everything and everyone is against you, you'll be defeated before you even begin. If you dwell in the doldrums and look down upon yourself and your body, why would your body work with you to help you heal? Instead, it's important to begin from a place of high self-esteem, with confidence and a capable, "can-do" attitude. Having high self-esteem means believing in yourself despite your current circumstances. Positive mantras can help point you in the right direction, and you don't need anyone or anything else to solidify those thoughts. This is not arrogance by any token; instead, it's simply believing that you are worth healing and happiness. (Newsflash: you are.)

You might have already had an inkling that how you feel about yourself will play into the overall success or failure of your healing. But there's another important component, and that is how you view the process of gut healing.

HOW YOU VIEW GUT HEALING

"This is too hard." "It's not worth it." "I am defeated already because everyone on my dad's side of the family has gut issues." "What's the point?"

Do any of those sound familiar? I'd love to tell you that I've never thought these things or said them out loud, but I have for sure. And when this was my mindset, I never healed. What I believed kept coming true, and what I told myself became my reality. Remember, if you don't actually make changes, nothing will change. If you stay stuck in a place of negativity about gut healing, nothing will change.

For every negative statement, there is an opposite thought or idea. When you begin to feel defeated, try replacing the negative thoughts with a positive one: "I've got this." "There is always something I can do to help my situation." "I will not give up." "There is so much hope." "I'm stronger than the circumstances." "Healing will happen." When I began to tell myself things like this and to replace my negative mindset, things began to change; I began to heal. No one ever said healing your gut would be easy, but if you believe you can and put in the work to make it happen, things will change.

In order to set yourself up for successful healing, you must possess a strong mindset about both yourself and the process. This won't work if you have high self-esteem but believe healing your gut is too hard. It also won't work if you tell yourself, "I've got this," but have a low sense of self-esteem. One of these alone isn't enough to initiate action. And action, darling, is the only way you can truly heal your gut.

MANTRAS TO HELP GET YOU STARTED

So, how do you begin to change your own mindset? I want to share some mantras to help get you started. I am so confident in the power of mantra

NOTES

I've made it a key part of the journaling process I recommend, as well as one of the Critical Actions you should be taking every day. The first thing you should do, before starting your journal, is to set a personal mantra, and begin saying it as often as possible.

To help you start, I've created a list of 31 gut-healing mantras. Some of these are mine that I have said over the years, while others I've collected from various sources. I want to give them all to you for inspiration.

1. My body is healthy; mind is brilliant; soul is tranquil.
2. I possess the qualities needed to be extremely successful.
3. My ability to conquer my challenges is limitless; my potential to succeed is infinite
4. I am at peace with all that has happened, is happening, and will happen.
5. Everything that is happening now is happening for my ultimate good.
6. I am a powerhouse; I am indestructible.
7. Though these times are difficult, they are only a short phase of life.
8. I am conquering my illness; I am defeating it steadily each day.
9. My life is just beginning.
10. Am I good enough? Yes, I am.
11. I'm allowed to take up space.

12. My past is not a reflection of my future.
13. Today I make the choices that allow me to thrive.
14. I am healed; I no longer have SIBO.
15. I am healing at my pace, not the pace from a book, magazine, or guru.
16. My body is healthy, and I'm grateful.
17. I'll surround myself with positive people who will help bring out the best in me.
18. I'm allowed to take the time to heal.
19. Perfection isn't the only way to success.
20. I accept the lesson my pain is offering me.
21. This illness doesn't define me.
22. Difficult times are part of my journey and allow me to appreciate the good.
23. This will be my healthiest year yet.
24. I let go of all that no longer serves me.
25. Negative thoughts only have the power I allow them.
26. My pain, both mental and physical, is gone.
27. Everything I am going through is making me a stronger, wiser, and more compassionate person.
28. I have created the perfect rainbow of health.
29. The bloat is gone, and I am free to live.
30. It is time to heal, and I choose to be in alignment with my body's way of doing that.
31. I honor my body's wisdom by trusting the signals that it sends.

You can use this list to help you get started, but I believe you should also create your own mantras based on your unique circumstances.

Right now, you could sink in and let your current circumstances take over, or you could get your mindset clear and right, plant those seeds, and watch as you bloom. Your mind is powerful. You are powerful.

CRITICAL ACTIONS TO TAKE TODAY:

- ☐ Get at least 8 hours of sleep.
- ☐ Record all bowel movements (time and type).
- ☐ Follow the "Say Yes" and "Say No" lists on pages 54–55 and 62–72.
- ☐ Choose meals from the Creations chapter on page 212.
- ☐ Record what you're eating—*all* the ingredients, not just the "ingredient(s)" (see page 103).
- ☐ Consume at least 8 cups of water.
- ☐ Write one line of gratitude and/or your healing mantra.
- ☐ Choose a workout activity that ranks no more than a 5 on an intensity scale of 1 to 10, and work out for a brief period of time.
- ☐ Do one thing your practitioner has told you to do but you just have not done yet.
- ☐ Record what cycle day (CD) you're on for your menstrual cycle (CD 1 = the day your period starts).

ACTIONS FOR YOU TO CONSIDER TAKING TODAY:

- ☐ Journal. What do you currently believe about your gut-healing journey?
- ☐ Make a list of *your* favorite mantras to start saying. Remember, they need to align with your personal circumstances. Bonus action: Do something creative with those mantras. For example, place them in strategic spots, like in your car, on your bathroom mirror, in your healing journal, etc.
- ☐ On a sheet of paper, write out the negative things you often find yourself saying. Then cross them out, one by one, and write words to replace them. Journal about the process, starting with, "When I crossed out the negative statement about why I could not heal my gut and replaced it with the positive statement, I felt . . ."

CREATION IDEAS FOR TODAY:

- ☐ Blackberry Salad Bowl (page 234)
- ☐ Harvest Bowl (page 236)
- ☐ Beef, Chicken, or Vegetable Broth (page 240)

GUT REAL THOUGHT FOR TODAY:

Health is not simply the absence of sickness.
—Hannah Green

NOTES

NOTES

The absence of sickness doesn't automatically mean we are healthy—slow leaks lead to flat tires. Your body is either a work in progression or regression. You can be in regression, even when you're "healthy," and you can be making progress, even when you're "sick."

When I first began writing about gut health, my goal was to help women with temporary issues. I knew that GI issues were on the rise, and I knew that there were women out there suffering just as I was, in silence. But what I did not expect was just how complicated these issues could be.

I thought IBS was IBS was IBS—in other words, those with IBS had similar symptoms that should be easy to overcome with a strict diet. Food was the medicine and the cure, and with this thinking, I would be able to help millions of women worldwide address their gut issues and move on with life.

How wrong I was.

At a very basic level, IBS certainly is not IBS is not IBS. In the years that followed, I found that this onion had layers to peel that I never knew existed. I began to study and understand that there were three pieces to most people's mysterious puzzles:

1. Diagnosis
2. Root causes
3. Triggers

You might think all three are one and the same, but in most cases, they are not. And healing your gut means learning about and addressing all three.

Let's look at a hypothetical example. Hope is not feeling well. She hasn't been feeling well for about 6 months. She's feeling more bloated

NOTES

by the day, but her bowel movements are inconsistent. She toggles between constipation and diarrhea, not knowing what might happen on any given day. Hope is also feeling more tired and seems to gain weight no matter what foods she eats or does not eat.

So Hope makes an appointment with her doctor. Dr. Rivers listens to her complaints and gets her set up with some lab work, including a CBC (complete blood count) and measuring her TSH (thyroid-stimulating hormone) levels. Hope gets the labs done that day and then goes home to wait for Dr. Rivers to call with answers.

But when Dr. Rivers calls, she says, "Your TSH levels are fine, CBC came back normal, and I'm suspecting IBS. Your **DIAGNOSIS** is IBS. IBS stands for irritable bowel syndrome," Dr. Rivers explains. "This means that you have a collective set of symptoms classified as a syndrome, not a disease." The conversation ends with a generic prescription for laxatives, over-the-counter medicines, and advice to "see if dairy affects how you feel."

Hope goes about her days. She tries some of the things Dr. Rivers mentioned, but things don't change. Another 6 months down the line, she finds herself feeling worse than ever, so she goes through doctor after doctor, step after step, until finally another doctor orders more tests, and then diagnoses her with SIBO (small intestinal bacterial overgrowth), a low-functioning thyroid, and a mild case of candida.

The SIBO, low-functioning thyroid, and candida are the **ROOT CAUSES** of the IBS diagnosis she was given years before.

With the help of her doctor, Hope begins implementing a healing protocol that includes dietary changes, a medication, and supplements. She feels grateful because she's *finally* feeling better.

But about 6 months later, all of a sudden, she starts not feeling optimal again. She doesn't understand why, and the words play in her head on repeat: "I'm following the diet, taking the medication, and keeping up with the supplements religiously. So why am I not feeling well? Now what?"

Hope begins to panic. She starts Googling every symptom she has. She convinces herself there is something else going on. (Spoiler alert: There is *nothing else* going on. Hope is, in fact, healing, slowly but surely.)

By this time, she's tired of going to the doctor, so she diagnoses herself with an underlying autoimmune condition. She concludes that she should diet harder with an AIP (autoimmune protocol) diet. Along with the diet, she introduces more supplements to the regimen. This healing process has now become Hope's full-time job; the cycle is ugly, hard, and both physically and mentally exhausting. And the new changes to her diet and supplements don't seem to be having any effect.

But remember when Hope first started not feeling well again? During that time, she was

NOTES

working late hours, was experiencing a rough patch with her husband, and, to help with all the stress, she was working out 5 days a week for 90 minutes per session.

When she wasn't feeling well, Hope thought about everything *but* lifestyle. But those lifestyle factors were **TRIGGERS**. A trigger can set you back, but a trigger does *not* mean you need to do more. In fact, as in Hope's case, it may mean you need to do less.

This story is a very common one. Because we place diagnosis, root causes, and triggers into one flowerpot, we expect that the same water will work for all of them in the same way. But they are not the same, and you will need to address each element in its own way in order to heal.

There are a few things I want you to take from Hope's story:

1. Understand that your diagnosis, root causes, and triggers are *not* one and the same.
2. Know that the right diagnosis, root cause(s), and triggers are *not* always easy to identify.
3. Accept that while your diagnosis and root cause(s) can typically be reached like a final destination, your triggers are different. Managing your own triggers is a lifelong journey you'll need to work on forever.

The good news is, armed with the information, assistance, and tools for self-empowerment in this bible, you are better equipped than ever before for the journey.

CRITICAL ACTIONS TO TAKE TODAY:

- ☐ Get at least 8 hours of sleep.
- ☐ Record all bowel movements (time and type).
- ☐ Follow the "Say Yes" and "Say No" lists on pages 54–55 and 62–72.
- ☐ Choose meals from the Creations chapter on page 212.
- ☐ Record what you're eating—*all* the ingredients, not just the "ingredient(s)" (see page 103).
- ☐ Consume at least 8 cups of water.
- ☐ Write one line of gratitude and/or your healing mantra.
- ☐ Choose a workout activity that ranks no more than a 5 on an intensity scale of 1 to 10, and work out for a brief period of time.
- ☐ Do one thing your practitioner has told you to do but you just have not done yet.
- ☐ Record what cycle day (CD) you're on for your menstrual cycle (CD 1 = the day your period starts).

ACTIONS FOR YOU TO CONSIDER TAKING TODAY:

- ☐ Journal. Are there ways in which you see yourself through the lens of Hope's story?
- ☐ Make three columns on a sheet of paper: one for Diagnosis, one for Root Causes, and one for Triggers. In each column, write down everything you *know for sure* (or have been told up

to this point) about each category. Look at the three columns. Ask yourself, in the most honest way possible, "Do I believe all of these to be true? What's missing?" Then, make a list of the action steps you'll take from those thoughts.

CREATION IDEAS FOR TODAY:

☐ Egg Roll Salad Bowl (page 234)

☐ Seafood or Fish Soup Bowl (page 243)

☐ Coconut-Honey Chicken (page 245)

GUT REAL THOUGHT FOR TODAY:

Did you know? According to the National Institutes of Health, "Women are up to two times more likely than men to develop IBS. People younger than age 50 are more likely to develop IBS than people older than age 50."[3]

---

[3]https://www.niddk.nih.gov/health-information/digestive-diseases/irritable-bowel-syndrome/definition-facts

After reading Hope's story yesterday, some of you might be thinking, *Okay, maybe this* **is** *all just in my head.*

NOTES

Please know that my intentions are always to lift you up so that you heal, and every last thing you are thinking and feeling is valid. While many people's stories end like Hope's story, sometimes there is also more to the root cause than was first discovered. If you have truly addressed all three pillars: diagnosis, diet, and lifestyle (see pages 22–23), and your gut is still telling you there's more to the story, please listen to your gut.

Honestly, our gut feelings are usually accurate, both in terms of our health and in other areas of life. When my gut instincts told me I should *not* be taking a new job, but I took it anyway, I ended up in court with a shady company over several months of not being paid. My gut instincts told me it was wrong to stay in a relationship with someone who always placed me last, but I stayed for years. Within a few months of finally leaving, I met my current husband. And my gut instincts told me that the diagnosis of IBS both my dad and I had received was BS. It took years, but eventually I was diagnosed with SIBO, a low-functioning thyroid, colitis, and adrenal fatigue, while my dad was diagnosed with stage 4 colon cancer.

So please believe me when I say that if your gut is telling you, "There's something more. Don't give up," you should listen. Do not stop with where you're at and what you've been told today.

That said, there is a fine line to walk when listening to your gut. For most of my life, I've been told I was a hypochondriac. And in some ways, it was true. I can't tell you the number of times I went to the nurse's office in elementary and middle school because I thought I was sick. I wasn't. I've gone into full panic attacks over simple things that had me convinced I was dying. So, yes, I have had tendencies toward hypochondria.

But as I got older and truly began having health issues, I still got told, "It's all in your mind." For the longest time I believed everyone, from family to friends to doctors. Deep down, I knew there had to be more to the story because I had very real external symptoms. Rash-like acne coated my face, and I could weigh 110 pounds and still look pregnant within 60 seconds of eating anything.

But because people told me it was in my head and I knew I had a past inclination toward hypochondria, I began believing perhaps even these physical manifestations were just in my own head.

So I stayed complacent. I was okay with the generic diagnosis I'd received, because I didn't want to make a big deal out of it. Instead of pursuing more tests and finding real answers, I internalized everything that was happening, turning more frequently to Dr. Google and becoming more scared and stressed as the years went by. And of course, in the meantime, my symptoms actually continued getting far worse.

By the time I received my real diagnoses, I had been straddling the line between listening to my gut and thinking, "Maybe it's all in my head," for so long that it was hard for me to know what was real and what was not. When friends and family members questioned my new diet protocols or asked questions about my diagnosis like, "Is this a credible doctor, or what?" I would do an internal eye roll, but a part of me would also think, "Wait, maybe this isn't legit?!"

Once, a family member asked me, "Are you really sick or are you just crazy?" I about lost it right then and there. With a lump in my throat and my body warm and tingling, I had to escape to my car to cry. In that moment, I wished I had my medical records to whip out of my purse, because I knew I was not crazy.

I often wonder why people feel they have the right to judge the way in which we live, or why my lifestyle would bother someone enough that snide comments roll off their tongue. After all, I don't go to friends' houses and question their lifestyles by saying, "Why are you eating McDonald's low-fat ice cream?" or "You complain about always feeling miserable, so maybe you should look at how you live your life." My eating or not eating asparagus, or apples, or anything else "normal" people deem as healthy quite obviously doesn't affect anyone but me, so I'm not sure why people feel the need to comment on it.

After that family member called me crazy, I seriously considered carrying my medical records in my already-too-cluttered purse. There would be no better way to prove what my blood tests

NOTES

had determined, and to say, "No, I am not crazy. I am just trying to get better."

But the truth is, no one really cares to see my medical records. They don't care about hearing that level of detail, and I don't need to prove myself to others, anyway. You owe no one any explanation for trying to heal.

There will always be others who are ready to judge your lifestyle. The line between trusting your gut and allowing your mind to play tricks on you will always be a fine one. But your gut is smart, and it's constantly speaking to you in one way or another. Choose to trust yourself and listen to it.

CRITICAL ACTIONS TO TAKE TODAY:

- ☐ Get at least 8 hours of sleep.
- ☐ Record all bowel movements (time and type).
- ☐ Follow the "Say Yes" and "Say No" lists on pages 54–55 and 62–72.
- ☐ Choose meals from the Creations chapter on page 212.
- ☐ Record what you're eating—*all* the ingredients, not just the "ingredient(s)" (see page 103).
- ☐ Consume at least 8 cups of water.
- ☐ Write one line of gratitude and/or your healing mantra.
- ☐ Choose a workout activity that ranks no more than a 5 on an intensity scale of 1 to 10, and work out for a brief period of time.
- ☐ Do one thing your practitioner has told you to do but you just have not done yet.
- ☐

☐ Record what cycle day (CD) you're on for your menstrual cycle (CD 1 = the day your period starts).

ACTIONS FOR YOU TO CONSIDER TAKING TODAY:

☐ Journal. Write about a time when you did not listen to your gut. What happened?

☐ Journal. Have you been questioned by anyone about anything on your journey? How does it make you feel?

☐ Think about the remarks people make about you, your journey, your decisions, your health, and so on. How do you want to respond when someone questions why you are doing things a certain way? Take the chance now to collect a list of responses, so that you're prepared next time this situation arises.

CREATION IDEAS FOR TODAY:

☐ Simple Salad Morning Bowl (page 230)

☐ Lamb Bowl (page 239)

☐ Wild Salmon (page 245)

GUT REAL THOUGHT FOR TODAY:

Don't confuse people who are always around you with people who are always there for you.

Not everyone is going to be supportive of the changes you are trying to make. Those who aren't supportive are perhaps those very same people you need to reconsider your relationship with

NOTES

going forward. Healing the gut and becoming truly healthy is also impacted by our relationships. Good relationships encourage us. They help us thrive. These are the relationships we need to help us grow.

You know how they say you can hear something a million times, but it isn't until the million and first time that it clicks in a whole new way? When I was a child and attending Catholic elementary school, I remember hearing repeatedly, "There is only one of you. No one else in the entire world is like you. Therefore you're special." It was easy for me to believe those words back then, and in many ways, I took them to heart. I believed that it was okay for me to be my own person, unlike anyone else.

But when I entered gut hell, I found that those words failed me. I never *truly* believed that **"If there is no one else like you in the world, then there is no one diet or way to heal your gut."**

In fact, I pushed against this idea as hard as I could for nearly my entire journey. I told myself that it simply could not be true: Paleo would work. Low-FODMAP was the answer. AIP really was miraculous. Carbohydrates would always be the enemy for everyone, no matter what.

After all, I thought, weren't we all human? I convinced myself that one after another of these one-size-fits all protocols was *the way* to forever healing, health, and happiness.

I took a dogmatic approach, fully adhering to whatever "rules" I was currently abiding by, because I believe that if it had worked for Sally Jane down the street, surely it would work the same for me.

Today, I look back on all that and I feel sad. Not just because it took me over a decade to finally get it, but because every single day I see these one-size-fits-all declarations everywhere I look. In the gut-healing community, I see people jumping on every bandwagon on the spectrum, from only eating meat to only eating vegetables; and from celebrating fiber as the solution for everyone to avoiding fiber at all costs. Out of a desperate desire to heal and to belong, we choose communities to align with and then stay so dedicated to them that we can't see any other perspective.

This is what leads people to argue and act in a superior manner to anyone whose staunch views don't align with their own. Oh, believe me, I have been there—I am as guilty of this as the next person, and I own up to it.

But darling, this is the truth that you need to hear today and that no other gut-health book out there will tell you:

There is no one else like you in the world.

Today, I have fully realized the power of these words, and I own them in a positive light to help women worldwide heal their guts, and their lives, on *their* terms.

What I could only wish I believed way back when is what I want you to believe today: If there is no one else like you in the world, then there is no one-size-fits-all diet or lifestyle that will heal your gut. There's only the way that's right for *you*.

CRITICAL ACTIONS TO TAKE TODAY:

☐ Get at least 8 hours of sleep.

- [ ] Record all bowel movements (time and type).
- [ ] Follow the "Say Yes" and "Say No" lists on pages 54–55 and 62–72.
- [ ] Choose meals from the Creations chapter on page 212.
- [ ] Record what you're eating—*all* the ingredients, not just the "ingredient(s)" (see page 103).
- [ ] Consume at least 8 cups of water.
- [ ] Write one line of gratitude and/or your healing mantra.
- [ ] Choose a workout activity that ranks no more than a 5 on an intensity scale of 1 to 10, and work out for a brief period of time.
- [ ] Do one thing your practitioner has told you to do but you just have not done yet.
- [ ] Record what cycle day (CD) you're on for your menstrual cycle (CD 1 = the day your period starts).

ACTIONS FOR YOU TO CONSIDER TAKING TODAY:

- [ ] Journal. Consider all the templated protocols you've tried on your journey that did *not* work for you. Dig deeper to understand why they didn't work for you.
- [ ] Think about something you are clinging to today and ask yourself, "Is this working for me?" If not, write it down and then consider letting it go. If and when you do let it go, also record that. In a couple weeks, see if letting go served you well.

NOTES

CREATION IDEAS FOR TODAY:

☐ Cucumber Bowl (page 231)

☐ Chicken and Squash Bowl (page 237)

☐ Berry-Licious Hemp Smoothie (page 219)

GUT REAL THOUGHT FOR TODAY:

Jet pilots don't have rearview mirrors.

My father-in-law passed this fact down to me, and I am passing it on to you: Jet pilots don't have rearview mirrors, and neither should you.

It's easy to get wrapped up in all the misery that came before, all the things you miss from before, or all the could've-should've-beens. But don't.

You are not the same person you were before you started this journey. You are shedding layers (physically and, hopefully, emotionally) that will no longer serve you in the future. Don't look back. Keep on preparing for all the awesome that lies ahead.

While there is not *one way* to eat for gut healing and gut health, there is *a way.* That way is the way you create, customized to and for you, and to and for you *only.*

You may be thinking, "So if the only way to eat is custom for me, then why do you have a 'Say Yes' and 'Say No' list in this book, and why are you recommending specific Creations for me each day?"

It's important to remember that these 21 days are only meant to be a starting point for your healing path. The plan you follow for these 21 days is not meant for you to carry on month after month.

Almost every single trustworthy medical source out there will tell you that any food elimination period should only last from 2 to 6 weeks. This 21-day program is meant to be a "phase 1" for your journey. This initial period is designed to help you begin to feel some relief, and to give you the ability to drill down further for identifying problematic foods. No phase 1 of an elimination diet is completely sane, nor is it optimal for an extended length of time—this is not meant to be a sustainable way of living over the long term; it's just your starting point.

The overall idea of phase 1 is to calm the digestive system down and reduce inflammation. This will enable you to effectively add foods back in, one at a time, to realize what truly is and is not working with your unique body composition.

I created the "Say Yes" and "Say No" lists to help guide you to the ingredients and whole foods that will help you achieve this goal. So many

NOTES

gut-health books out there are filled with recipes, but don't offer detailed guidance on the individual ingredients that will and will not work for an elimination diet. While I enjoy trying new recipes, my healing success required an understanding of the single-ingredient foods that were and were not working for me along the way, so that I could take those foods and customize my own meals from them. I've provided you with the "Yes" and "No" lists to empower you to do the same.

I've also offered you "Creation" ideas for each day, rather than more traditional recipes, for two reasons. First, I wanted to give you ample ideas for what to eat and inspire you to customize your meals to suit your own taste and your own dietary requirements. But the Creation ideas were also created with minimal ingredients so you will be able to easily track any reactions over the course of your 21 days.

I truly believe that if you have never tried changing your diet and lifestyle to help with your lingering gut issues, this is the perfect place to start. But I also believe that if you have no answers after these 21 days, then dieting harder is definitely *not* your answer.

In my case, for example, even one of the most stringent protocols out there, the GAPS (gut and psychology syndrome) diet, did not bring me long-term healing, because it wasn't addressing my real underlying issues. Dieting harder would have never gotten me to the SIBO answer—only testing could do that. If a gut-healing protocol or diet helps you feel better, then you know you're on to something. But if it doesn't, dieting harder is not going to solve every outstanding problem. Remember, if you haven't been appropriately tested, then dieting harder makes no sense. The point of a diet is to solve a problem, and if you don't know the problem, you can't solve it. And once you do know the problem you're trying to solve, diet, while critical for healing, will be far from the only healing variable. You'll also need to look at your stress levels, physical activity, sleep, relationships, skincare products, environment, and so much more. Your dieting willpower will not be "the one thing" in the end that makes or breaks your path to long-lasting healing. If simply dieting harder were the answer, almost everyone would be healed.

Remember, this is meant for 21 days. Stick to it.

CRITICAL ACTIONS TO TAKE TODAY:

☐ Get at least 8 hours of sleep.

☐ Record all bowel movements (time and type).

☐ Follow the "Say Yes" and "Say No" lists on pages 54–55 and 62–72.

☐ Choose meals from the Creations chapter on page 212.

☐ Record what you're eating—*all* the ingredients, not just the "ingredient(s)" (see page 103).

☐ Consume at least 8 cups of water.

☐ Write one line of gratitude and/or your healing mantra.

NOTES

NOTES

☐ Choose a workout activity that ranks no more than a 5 on an intensity scale of 1 to 10, and work out for a brief period of time.

☐ Do one thing your practitioner has told you to do but you just have not done yet.

☐ Record what cycle day (CD) you're on for your menstrual cycle (CD 1 = the day your period starts).

ACTIONS FOR YOU TO CONSIDER TAKING TODAY:

☐ Journal. What do you believe about diets as they relate to your healing journey? Really explore those thoughts. If you are tied to any specific way of dieting for healing, keep asking yourself, "Why am I tied to this?" Dig even deeper, asking, "If I'm so tied to this way of eating for healing, then why am I still not feeling well?"

☐ Do you have a list of foods that you know, for sure, without a doubt, work for you? If so, make a list of these foods and keep it in your food journal.

CREATION IDEAS FOR TODAY:

☐ Bacon Bowl (page 228)

☐ Apricot Chicken (page 244)

☐ Coconutty Smoothie (page 219)

GUT REAL THOUGHT FOR TODAY:

When you have the will, you always have the way.

There are countless ways we pave the way for the things we wish to bring alive in life. Healing your gut is no different. If you have the will, you will find the way. I made excuses for years because I didn't have the will, until finally, enough was enough. If you've purchased this book, you've probably found that enough is enough for you as well. You have the will. Now you just need to find your way.

NOTES

NOTES

Yesterday we talked about how food elimination will factor into your success, and why I've offered you suggested Creations for each of these 21 days. But it's important to note that what I have outlined for the 21 days of food *still* might not be for you. (Remember, you are not a pastry—there is no mold that will perfectly fit you!) Therefore, many of the Creation ideas on page 212 include additional customization options. This was done very intentionally, because while I want to provide you with clear, easy-to-follow guidelines, I *also* want to provide you the freedom to step outside the guidelines when you need to.

Already diagnosed with SIBO, not currently on an antibiotic, and your doctor has advised you to remain low-FODMAP? Alright, then don't eat the avocado.

Recently diagnosed with diverticulitis and your doctor is telling you, "Less fats and animal-based products; more fiber"? Well, then great, some of the Creations would pair nicely with a brown rice. Go for it!

I could give a hundred examples like this, but the bottom line is that you must listen to your own body first and foremost. And I'm not just talking about these 21 days, but for the rest of your life.

CRITICAL ACTIONS TO TAKE TODAY:
☐ Get at least 8 hours of sleep.
☐ Record all bowel movements (time and type).
☐ Follow the "Say Yes" and "Say No" lists on pages 54–55 and 62–72.

☐ Choose meals from the Creations chapter on page 212.

☐ Record what you're eating—*all* the ingredients, not just the "ingredient(s)" (see page 103).

☐ Consume at least 8 cups of water.

☐ Write one line of gratitude and/or your healing mantra.

☐ Choose a workout activity that ranks no more than a 5 on an intensity scale of 1 to 10, and work out for a brief period of time.

☐ Do one thing your practitioner has told you to do but you just have not done yet.

☐ Record what cycle day (CD) you're on for your menstrual cycle (CD 1 = the day your period starts).

ACTIONS FOR YOU TO CONSIDER TAKING TODAY:

☐ Journal. Think about a gut-healing diet or, various diets, you've tried that did not work for you. Recall what it was like to follow the template and unpack why you suspect it did not work. Were there pieces that possibly worked? If so, what were they?

☐ Try making your *own* Creation today! Choose ingredients already included in the Creations on pages 212–251, and/or on the "Say Yes" list on pages 54–55. What did you make? Did you enjoy the process and outcome?

NOTES

CREATION IDEAS FOR TODAY:

☐ Breakfast Fruit Bowl (page 228)

☐ Duck Bowl (page 237)

☐ Herbed Burger (page 246)

GUT REAL THOUGHT FOR TODAY:

Just because fruits and veggies are "good for us" doesn't mean they are all good for us. Review the information on saccharides on page 258, and be truthful with yourself. Are you eating a ton of fruit and vegetables? Revisit your journals. Find patterns. And remember, this is just one example: The patterns affecting your own gut health might not be about fruits and vegetables. Your own patterns are just that—your own. We are creatures of habit, though, so if you are feeling miserable, there is likely a trail that could lead you to some answers.

For many years, I proudly preached a doctrine of "food and lifestyle, not drugs and medications." If you want the truth, I felt a sort of superiority about doing it all unmedicated, and the ideas I heard from my alternative practitioners and friends only fueled my fire.

The problem was, while I was preaching this message of food and lifestyle alone, I never fully healed. In the end, it took a combination of antibiotics and medications prescribed over the course of a few years, including low-dose naltrexone (LDN), WP Thyroid, rifaximin, and neomycin, to finally help me fully heal. And even after my gut symptoms had begun to heal, I found that there was still a place for medication in maintaining my overall health.

I'll never forget the fateful day in early fall 2018 when I went on an outing with my cousin and my three kids, who were 2, 3, and 4 years old at the time. There was a corn maze, a corn pit, food, and hayrides, and so many laughs and smiling faces. But there I was, in the middle of this huge place, feeling so much anxiety and so many pent-up emotions. I snapped at everyone and everything all day. While on the hayride, I cried. Tears fell under my shaded glasses, and my heart ached for reasons I could not understand or express. Shortly after the hayride, I loaded up the kids for the hour-long drive home. And on that drive, I pondered the gut-brain axis. (I mean, isn't this what everyone does when they can't understand their emotions?!) What I could not understand

NOTES

was how, with my gut finally the best it had ever been—I had just had a perfect colonoscopy and endoscopy—I still felt so *off* in my mind. I knew there had to be more going on.

When I got home, my husband took the kids and I retreated to our room. My mind was exhausted from the overwhelming emotions that had finally erupted that day. I lay in bed, crying without fully understanding why, and vowed that something *would* change.

The very next day, I finally made a long-overdue appointment to see a doctor. This time, I went the Western-medicine route, because it was different than anything I had previously tried. (Remember, nothing changes if nothing changes!) Fortunately, the doctor I saw that day was a woman who not only listened to me for a long time, even through my tears, but also empathized with my words. It was clear to her immediately that I had tried everything I could from a natural standpoint and had exhausted all the lifestyle options, so we discussed the idea of a medication for depression and anxiety called fluoxetine.

Previously, my gut instinct had always told me, "No medications for this." But that day, I told her I would gladly accept the prescription, along with a referral to a good therapist.

Within a week, I was on fluoxetine and had had my initial visit with the therapist. Since then, my life has dramatically improved for the better. I still take the medication *and* see the therapist, and my gut health is still in great shape, with no relapses.

While medication worked for me, that doesn't mean it will necessarily be the right choice for you. But I share this side of my healing story to show that sometimes, it's necessary to step outside of your self-imposed limits and try something new to make a change.

There will always be some experts who believe medicine is the ultimate destroyer of gut health, while others will say, "Medicine is the only thing that works; stop lying and recommending diet and lifestyle cures."

My truth, though, is that straddling the line between Western and alternative thinking was the key to my own healing. And I believe that if more health and wellness experts also straddled this line, far more of us could find happiness and true, lasting healing.

CRITICAL ACTIONS TO TAKE TODAY:

- ☐ Get at least 8 hours of sleep.
- ☐ Record all bowel movements (time and type).
- ☐ Follow the "Say Yes" and "Say No" lists on pages 54–55 and 62–72.
- ☐ Choose meals from the Creations chapter on page 212.
- ☐ Record what you're eating—*all* the ingredients, not just the "ingredient(s)" (see page 103). Consume at least 8 cups of water.
- ☐ Write one line of gratitude and/or your healing mantra.

NOTES

- ☐ Choose a workout activity that ranks no more than a 5 on an intensity scale of 1 to 10, and work out for a brief period of time.
- ☐ Do one thing your practitioner has told you to do but you just have not done yet.
- ☐ Record what cycle day (CD) you're on for your menstrual cycle (CD 1 = the day your period starts).

ACTIONS FOR YOU TO CONSIDER TAKING TODAY:

- ☐ Journal. Think about something, anything, in your life that you have been resisting due to one fear or another. How has this been holding you back? If you have let it hold you back for far too long, write out your ideas for how you can change today. What will you do? How will you make it happen?
- ☐ Journal. What are your thoughts about taking medications? (By the way, your thoughts are not right or wrong. Just be aware of what they are, why you have them, and whether the ideas you have today are the same as those you've had in the past. Do you think you'll continue to hold these same ideas in the future?)

CREATION IDEAS FOR TODAY:

- ☐ Nutty Bowl (page 229)
- ☐ Bacon Bowl (page 228)
- ☐ Turkey Patties (page 246)

GUT REAL THOUGHT FOR TODAY:

Does a sweet tooth have you down today? If so, just add a little honey or maple syrup to your diet. It should do the trick, and your gut will probably be okay with it. Here are a few suggestions for how to enjoy your sweet treat:

1. Put a little in your coffee with your coconut milk.
2. Drizzle it over fruit.
3. Stir some into your tea.
4. Whip it with full-fat coconut milk for a sweet dessert whipped topping.
5. Mix some into a salad dressing.

NOTES

NOTES

By this point in the 21-day process, hopefully you've gotten into the habit of writing in your journal each day. If you haven't, I urge you to start today! Journaling for gut healing is so important because it helps you to see where you've been and where you are. And if you don't know where you are at, then how will you know where you're going?

It's like driving a car: If you are driving somewhere and get lost, do you just continue wandering, hoping that you'll end up back on the correct path? No, you open your Google Maps app, and you make sure you are headed in the right direction! Otherwise, you know you'll lose time, become stressed, and likely never reach your destination. If you are awful with directions like me, you will get lost from time to time, but you never accept getting lost as your destination.

In a similar way, you never want to simply accept getting lost on your gut-healing journey. If you find you've gone down a wrong path, you need to check your map, so to speak, and get yourself back on track. This is why journaling is so effective.

Your journal will help you to visualize your healing and health story. It's your road map for where you are today, where you will go tomorrow, and where you want to be 3 months down the line. Without it, it will be hard to make impactful changes.

Here are a few of the ways journaling can help you heal your gut:

1. **Identifying Patterns:** Journaling will help you to better identify patterns in your digestive health. Looking over the history of the foods you're eating and how you're feeling can help you make correlations between food and your mood, food and your digestive symptoms, and food and your other symptoms.

2. **Processing Your Emotions:** I can't emphasize this enough: If you don't address every single emotion you're feeling, you might never fully heal. Journaling can help you to process and release the emotions that may be holding you back from making a change.

3. **Quieting Your Mind:** Once you're able to transfer the thoughts swirling inside your own head onto paper, your mind will become quieter. And when your mind becomes quieter, you are better able to process your own emotions (see #2).

4. **Finding Gratitude:** Healing will happen faster if you can focus on the positive, rather than the negative. When you feel your mindset heading downward in a negative direction, you can always attempt to turn it around by listing all the things you're grateful for in your journal. Sometimes simply writing them down can help you to see how much there is to be grateful for, and gratitude breeds more gratitude.

5. **Reflecting:** If you're journaling daily, I recommend keeping those journals year

after year so that you can look back and reflect on the path you've traveled so far. You'll be able to see where you were compared to where you are now, and where you still might need to go on your healing journey.

6. **Embracing Creativity:** Some of you might not care about this, but for many of us, finding a beautiful journal, getting some lovely pens or markers, and exploring our lives in a creative way can be such an inspiring tool for the healing journey.

I also want to remind you that wherever you are in this healing process, journaling remains an important part of the work you're doing. If you're still just getting started and don't yet have an accurate diagnosis, your journal can be helpful in giving you a baseline to start from.

It will allow you to give your doctor(s) and nutritionist(s) the concrete information and evidence they'll need to get you the right tests and find your correct diagnosis.

If you've been trying for a while to heal your gut without journaling consistently, but are having a hard time pinpointing the right strategy, it could be because everything you're doing is strictly based off memory. And guess what? If your gut is not well, brain fog could be getting the best of that beautiful mind. It's way too hard to try to manage your gut health from memory. If you find yourself not feeling well one evening, you may say, "Well, I think I had chicken, sweet potatoes, butter, red peppers, and dark chocolate today," but with zero context about anything else, it will be hard to identify what exactly is triggering your symptoms. Your chances of hitting a target with a blindfold on are slim. And if you're working with a medical practitioner to manage your symptoms, it can be helpful for both of you to keep all the relevant information in one organized place.

You may find that journaling helps you identify patterns beyond your gut, as well. Remember, 70 to 90% of our immune system cells lie within the gut, whatever other conditions you're dealing with, they likely have roots within the gut. Hormonal issues, infertility, skin conditions, anxiety . . . keeping track of your day-to-day choices and symptoms can help with managing all these conditions, and many more.

Finally, if you have, or suspect you have, a Gutsy child, journaling can be a great tool for you to use as a mama bear to help navigate your child's health. I've been there, too, with my son, and I can't tell you how helpful it can be to keep your thoughts organized in a journal as you work on building your children's microbiomes.

Whether you use these pages, my *Healing Blooms from Within* journal, or your own favorite notebook or phone app, get in the journaling habit to help you take control of the situation before it takes control of you.

NOTES

CRITICAL ACTIONS TO TAKE TODAY:

☐ Get at least 8 hours of sleep.

☐ Record all bowel movements (time and type).

☐ Follow the "Say Yes" and "Say No" lists on pages 54–55 and 62–72.

☐ Choose meals from the Creations chapter on page 212.

☐ Record what you're eating—*all* the ingredients, not just the "ingredient(s)" (see page 103).

☐ Consume at least 8 cups of water.

☐ Write one line of gratitude and/or your healing mantra.

☐ Choose a workout activity that ranks no more than a 5 on an intensity scale of 1 to 10, and work out for a brief period of time.

☐ Do one thing your practitioner has told you to do but you just have not done yet.

☐ Record what cycle day (CD) you're on for your menstrual cycle (CD 1 = the day your period starts).

ACTIONS FOR YOU TO CONSIDER TAKING TODAY:

☐ Journal. What has journaling taught you so far? If you still haven't started journaling, take a piece of paper and simply write out the reasons why you don't want to journal. Tell yourself why you don't think it's useful and why it can't help you on your journey. Then reread your list and ask yourself, "Are these thoughts and ideas prohibiting me from healing?"

☐ You've been recording all bowel movements

for at least 11 days now. Are you starting to see any patterns? What are you seeing about them that you might not have noticed without meticulously tracking?

CREATION IDEAS FOR TODAY:

- ☐ Packed Protein Bowl (page 239)
- ☐ Berries 'n' Greens Smoothie (page 219)
- ☐ Turkey Legs with Brussels Sprouts and Raisins (page 245)

GUT REAL THOUGHT FOR TODAY:

Pearls do not lie on the seashore. If you desire one, you must dive for it. —Ancient Proverb

What we truly desire, we will dive for no matter what. I used to believe that "All good things come to those who wait." But I've realized that this is almost never true. The truth is good things come to those who work hard, not to those who wait.

If you're waiting for your gut to heal itself or for your lifestyle to transform into a healthier one, you'll likely wait forever. The body is brilliant, but neglecting it will get you nowhere. Working hard to keep it running as it should will yield huge benefits.

Continue diving in, and you'll see. If you're feeling miserable today, remember that after the rain comes the rainbow. I know you'll find yours, darling.

NOTES

Some things are just meant to go together: fall and pumpkin spice, summer and umbrella drinks, chocolate and strawberries, babies and puppies, Johnny and June, Thelma and Louise (am I dating myself here?!), cream and sugar. And some things, like peanut butter and jelly, not only go together, but they also physically stick together.

The same thing happens with gut issues—they are often so closely related to other health issues that they're deeply entwined, stuck together just like the PB&J on a sandwich. Some of the most common gut connections are:

1. Gut-liver
2. Gut-toxins
3. Gut–emotional issues
4. Gut–leaky gut
5. Gut–nutrition
6. Gut–digestive enzymes
7. Gut–immune system
8. Gut–stomach acid
9. Gut–mineral status
10. Gut–vagus nerve
11. Gut-thyroid
12. Gut–microbiome
13. Gut–gut infections
14. Gut-stress

Because the gut is so closely entwined with all these other systems, it's rare for gut issues to cause just one symptom. Instead, they can tend to cause a snowball effect. One thing happens, and then if that first issue is not addressed, the issues begin to snowball, with additional problems piling on and worsening the effects of the first issue. Eventually, the snowball becomes so large, the web of illness so entangled, that the issues are hard to separate.

The gut connections listed above can lead to hundreds of different medical conditions in countless combinations. Here are some of the most common ones to be aware of:

1. Allergies/asthma
2. Barrett's esophagus
3. Candida
4. Celiac disease
5. Chronic fatigue syndrome (CFS)
6. *Clostridium difficile*
7. Constipation
8. Crohn's disease
9. Diarrhea
10. Diverticulitis
11. *Escherichia coli*
12. Gastroesophageal reflux (GER) + gastroesophageal reflux disease (GERD)
13. Gallstones
14. Gastroenteritis (stomach flu)
15. Gluten sensitivity
16. *Helicobacter pylori*
17. Hemorrhoids
18. Hormone issues
19. Irritable bowel syndrome (IBS)
20. Lactose intolerance

NOTES

21. Leaky gut syndrome
22. Migraines
23. Pancreatitis
24. Parasites
25. Perioral dermatitis/other skin conditions
26. Small intestinal bacterial overgrowth (SIBO)
27. Stomach cancer
28. Stomach ulcers
29. Thyroid issues
30. Ulcerative colitis

I'm not telling you this to scare you, but because I want to encourage you to take control of your gut issues before they snowball too far out of control. If you are already experiencing the snowball effect, don't despair—it happened to me, too, and I am healed to an optimal place today. What you need to remember is that the longer you wait to take control of your life and health, the more the snowball grows out of control. If your doctor only does a standard CBC (complete blood count), and then sends you on your way with a "good bill of health" while you stay miserable, don't settle for that! Educate yourself about how your gut is connected to the rest of your bodily symptoms, and then advocate for the answers and solutions you need.

CRITICAL ACTIONS TO TAKE TODAY:
- ☐ Get at least 8 hours of sleep.
- ☐ Record all bowel movements (time and type).
- ☐ Follow the "Say Yes" and "Say No" lists on pages 54–55 and 62–72.

☐ Choose meals from the Creations chapter on page 212.

☐ Record what you're eating—*all* the ingredients, not just the "ingredient(s)" (see page 103).

☐ Consume at least 8 cups of water.

☐ Write one line of gratitude and/or your healing mantra.

☐ Choose a workout activity that ranks no more than a 5 on an intensity scale of 1 to 10, and work out for a brief period of time.

☐ Do one thing your practitioner has told you to do but you just have not done yet.

☐ Record what cycle day (CD) you're on for your menstrual cycle (CD 1 = the day your period starts).

ACTIONS FOR YOU TO CONSIDER TAKING TODAY:

☐ Journal. Think about the snowball effect as it relates to any piece of your life. It might be how one health issue has led to the next, *or* it might be how one decision you made has led to another. What has the snowball effect meant for your own life? And better yet, how can you melt the snow to heal the situation(s)?

☐ Look at the gut connections and medical connections lists above. Do you see yourself in any of those? Or are there any that you had *not* yet considered?

CREATION IDEAS FOR TODAY:

☐ Breakfast Fruit Bowl (page 228)

NOTES

☐ Roast Beef Bowl (page 237)

☐ Pineapple Salmon (page 245)

GUT REAL THOUGHT FOR TODAY:

It's only boring if you tell yourself it's boring.

Does "boring food" have you in the doldrums today? Let's address it.

Tough love: Your food is only boring if you tell yourself it's boring. Food doesn't have to be sexy to be enjoyable. It doesn't have to look like it came straight out of Martha Stewart's kitchen. It doesn't have to come in pink wrappers. It doesn't have to be smothered with frosting or heavy sauces. Society—and Pinterest—would have us believe that those are the only foods that are fun and taste good, but that simply isn't true. (And for the record, there's plenty of stunning-looking food on Pinterest that is also healing!)

I get that you may feel like you're stuck in a monotonous rut. Please remember that this process is not a lifelong diet—it's a bridge intended to simply reset your body, so you can begin adding all the other foods back in to find out what you can and cannot tolerate.

And I promise you, there is *no food* that tastes as good as a thriving gut feels. If your stomach has been in digestive hell for years, "boring" food might not seem so boring anymore when you remember the alternative. Remember, we all make choices . . . and then those choices ulti-mately make us.

I've always enjoyed working out, but I was never too serious about it . . . that is, until I moved to California. Maybe it was the year-round warm weather, the healthier-living scenery, or just the fact that I was prepping for my wedding around that time, but whatever the reason, I started working out a *ton*, in ways I never had before.

While in high school my friends had joked that I ran like an elephant (was it because of the way my feet waddled, or because I was slower than molasses?), when I took up long-distance running in California, I became fairly good at it. In fact, I ran my very first half-marathon ever in 1:48, feeling leaps and bounds more athletic than I had ever been in my entire life.

But I didn't stop there—I kept seeking out new and exciting ways to make my body as athletic as it could become. I ran short and long distance, lifted weights, did CrossFit-style workouts, and completed fitness program after program. At one point I even considered training for a Bikini Competition!

Even after I got sick, I *still* kept up with all of this. I didn't want to give it up, and I thought of working out as a necessary way to release all the stress that came with illness. Also, in my mind I thought, "Maybe if I just work out a little harder, the bloating will vanish."

I was desperate to both heal my gut and train like an Olympic athlete, and it took *years* before I realized that I had adopted conflicting goals: When you're constantly running and working out, your body is under a ton of stress. And when your body is under this amount of intense stress, it goes into fight-or-flight mode. It prioritizes "running from the bear" instead of digesting your food.

To fully heal, I had to take a mammoth step back and ask myself, "What for?" What am I working out like this for? Am I going to the Olympics? Will I ever win a half-marathon or set a record of any sort? When I was able to truly reflect on those questions and the answers they held, I saw how damaging those workouts were for my gut. As I began on my final steps toward true healing, I brought my workouts down to nothing. Yes, nothing. After doing absolutely nothing for quite some time, I began again with easy walking, and I stayed there for quite some time. In fact, I *still* do a lot of easy walking to this day, because working out with that level of minimalism changed my life.

And while this book is not about weight loss, and healing does not always equal losing weight, I would not be telling you the full story if I didn't tell you this: When my gut was desperate to heal, the less I worked out, the faster I got to my ideal weight, the weight where my body naturally wanted to be.

If you're used to working out intensely or giving a lot of thought to body aesthetics, it can be *hard* to break up with that mindset. I get it, believe me. And I'm not saying that you can't do intense workouts if you're feeling great. Just remember, conflicting goals will never get you to where you want to ultimately be.

CRITICAL ACTIONS TO TAKE TODAY:

- ☐ Get at least 8 hours of sleep.
- ☐ Record all bowel movements (time and type).
- ☐ Follow the "Say Yes" and "Say No" lists on pages 54–55 and 62–72.
- ☐ Choose meals from the Creations chapter on page 212.
- ☐ Record what you're eating—*all* the ingredients, not just the "ingredient(s)" (see page 103).
- ☐ Consume at least 8 cups of water.
- ☐ Write one line of gratitude and/or your healing mantra.
- ☐ Choose a workout activity that ranks no more than a 5 on an intensity scale of 1 to 10, and work out for a brief period of time.
- ☐ Do one thing your practitioner has told you to do but you just have not done yet.
- ☐ Record what cycle day (CD) you're on for your menstrual cycle (CD 1 = the day your period starts).

ACTIONS FOR YOU TO CONSIDER TAKING TODAY:

- ☐ Journal. What do your workouts consist of? Look back through the workouts you've been doing these past several days. Have you been choosing a workout activity that ranks no more than a 5 on an intensity scale of 1 to 10? If so, check in with yourself. Is this working for you, or is a 5 still too much?
- ☐ If you don't want to give up intense work-outs, take the time to explore *why*. Consider

spending even just 1 week doing nothing but leisure walking, biking, and/or stretching. Then write about what happened.

CREATION IDEAS FOR TODAY:

- ☐ Squash Breakfast Bowl (page 230)
- ☐ Chili Bowl (page 239)
- ☐ Build-Your-Own Smoothie Bowl (page 232)

GUT REAL THOUGHT FOR TODAY:

"What's going on inside of you, Jay? What are you afraid of? You've got a chance to change everything. Take it. This is about more than just surfing. This is about choices you make in life. This is about finding that one thing that sets you free. You need to believe in yourself or none of this matters." —Frosty, Chasing Mavericks

When I watched the movie *Chasing Mavericks*, I was struck by this quote. Like Jay's character in the movie, at any given moment, you also have the chance to change everything. This 21-day process is about more than just a diet; it's about the choices you make in life. These choices are not just a conscious decision regarding real or fake food. These choices include all aspects of your life, including both diet and lifestyle. It's about believing in and loving yourself enough to make the right decisions for healing and growth.

Something most people find a little shocking about me is that I was the ice hockey goalie in high school. Now, let me be clear: I was not good, not even a little bit. I did have one spectacular save, when the opposing team got a penalty shot—in other words, it was just one of their girls against me in the net. I will never in my life forget that save. She shot, and I went down almost into butterfly position, but as I went down, I watched the puck fly through the air to my left side and raised my glove hand in the air to catch the puck. To this day, I can feel the tug of the puck nestled in the net of my glove, shutting out that goal.

Other than that one shining moment, though, I was not any good at playing goalie.

So how did I end up as goalie in the first place? After about 10 years of practicing gymnastics, as a ninth grader I was *tired* of the mind games gymnastics played with me. Some of my best friends were on the hockey team, so one day I just up and quit gymnastics and headed straight for the ice rink. I started as a wing, usually left wing, and I wasn't much good at this position, either. But I had a great attitude, I'll tell you that. So when our one and only goalie told the coach, with only about a week's notice, that she would be gone for the holiday tournament my sophomore year, and Coach asked, "Well, does anyone want to take a shot in the net?" I fearlessly raised my hand and said, without hesitation, "I will."

I figured, what did I have to lose? I wasn't that good at playing wing anyway, and if I didn't like it, I would just return to wing after the holiday tournament. I took a leap of faith, and I was given the job.

I had just *two* practices before the tournament to learn how to wear goalie skates and put on all the bulky, unfamiliar gear. In fact, the first time I stood in full gear, I could hardly skate. I looked like Bambi, hobbling and wobbling around. Nonetheless, the very first game found me standing in front of the net, ready to take on an incredibly difficult team. I took shot after shot and watched as puck after puck flew into my net. One, two, three, five, ten, twelve goals later, and the nightmare still wasn't over. I grew weary, was totally embarrassed, and felt completely *crushed*.

But I stayed in the net for all three periods. At the end of the game, our team had lost 19–0.

Yes, you're reading that correctly. And yes, I did say hockey, not basketball. The score was 19–0.

There were many tears shed that night, and a lot of concerns knowing that I still had two more games to make it through that weekend. My team lost the next game 11–2, and the final game, we lost just 4–1.

When it was over, I didn't want to leave the position. Our goalie came back, but I stayed put as the backup goalie. I practiced the rest of the season in the net. I would be on one side of the rink, and she would be on the other side. I was okay with the fact that I might not play the rest of the year, because I had finally found a position that worked for me.

It worked for me because I loved the challenge of stopping as many pucks as I could. I'm not sure I would have stayed with hockey for the rest of high school had I not accidentally stumbled into the goalie position. If they had asked me even 2 weeks before the tournament about taking the goalie position on, I would have said, "No way. I've never done it. I don't know how to do it, and it wouldn't work for me."

But I stepped outside my comfort zone, and in the process, I found one of the best things that would happen for me throughout high school.

So, what does this have to do with gut healing?

Everything. Years later, while working with my very first nutritionist, I had a similar experience of how helpful it can be to step outside the box sometimes.

After a food intolerance test showed that I was intolerant to 22 foods, the nutritionist put me on a fairly strict, mostly vegetarian, diet. It worked okay at first—the diet was far healthier than the packaged foods and dairy I had been eating previously, so I did feel somewhat better. But after a short amount of time, I was back to feeling pretty miserable with bloat and constipation. As I started doing my own research, I stumbled upon the GAPS (gut and psychology syndrome) Diet by Dr. Natasha Campbell-McBride. It was the opposite of what I had been doing, which was consuming nearly no animal products and minimal fat. But my gut instincts told me, "Make a complete 180, do it for a little bit, and see what happens. You

NOTES

have nothing to lose." I brought the idea to the nutritionist, and she agreed it couldn't hurt to try an equal yet opposite approach.

That decision, that directional change, sent me on my forever-healing path. For my whole life I had been eating fat-free, sugar-free, and low-calorie foods, with minimal animal-based products, because that's what I believed would work. But I had to step out of that box to begin my healing journey. As with hockey, if I hadn't had the desire to try something new, I would have never stumbled upon something great.

This concept is a hard one for many women to understand. The idea of swapping a vegan diet for an animal-based one (or, on the flip side, of changing from a heavily animal-based diet to a vegan one) is completely out of the question for them. But remember, if the diet you're currently on isn't working, you *cannot fix the problem by dieting harder*. Sometimes, finding the answers requires a completely opposite approach. This isn't easy, but it may be the answer you needed to hear today.

CRITICAL ACTIONS TO TAKE TODAY:

☐ Get at least 8 hours of sleep.

☐ Record all bowel movements (time and type).

☐ Follow the "Say Yes" and "Say No" lists on pages 54–55 and 62–72.

☐ Choose meals from the Creations chapter on page 212.

☐ Record what you're eating—*all* the ingredients, not just the "ingredient(s)" (see page 103).

☐ Consume at least 8 cups of water.

☐ Write one line of gratitude and/or your healing mantra.

☐ Choose a workout activity that ranks no more than a 5 on an intensity scale of 1 to 10, and work out for a brief period of time.

☐ Do one thing your practitioner has told you to do but you just have not done yet.

☐ Record what cycle day (CD) you're on for your menstrual cycle (CD 1 = the day your period starts).

ACTIONS FOR YOU TO CONSIDER TAKING TODAY:

☐ Journal. What is one way you might be able to step out of a familiar box?

☐ Write about a correlation from something in your past to your current healing journey. You might uncover something about your-self or your tendencies that you never have previously.

CREATION IDEAS FOR TODAY:

☐ Papaya Sunrise Bowl (page 229)

☐ Wild Salmon and Hempseed Cauliflower Rice Bowl (page 236)

☐ Tomato Basil Chicken (page 244)

GUT REAL THOUGHT FOR TODAY:

Start Here: If you desire a glorious future, transform the present. —Patanjali

Day 14 means that you are just *1 week* away from the end! Can you believe it?

With just 1 week left, you should start to think about day 22 and beyond. You have already begun to transform your life, but even once these 21 days are over, I would encourage you to not give up and go back to all your "old ways." Starts and stops make the path to success much longer and more frustrating than it needs to be.

When I first tried a 21-day elimination diet, as the 22nd day approached, I was overwhelmed with excitement about transitioning back into a "normal" eating lifestyle. My first thought was, "Let's celebrate!"

I chose to reward myself with food, and that night, a bunch of us went out to dinner. I remember wanting to still stay focused, so I ordered fish and veggies—but also mashed potatoes loaded with butter and sour cream. For 20 minutes afterward, I was fine. Then, I started to get hot—really hot. My stomach felt horrible. I got sick, and my stomach continued to hurt, but everyone I was with wanted to go out for a drink. Thinking the sickness would pass, I agreed. As soon as we got to the bar, though, I was back in the bathroom. This time it was much worse. I was on my hands and knees, throwing up and sweating. I had to ask my cousin to take me home.

The next day, I felt fine. I never made the correlation between having "treated myself" that night and how sick I became, and on Day 23, I went back to eating my low-point Weight Watchers® processed garbage. Unsurprisingly, the vicious cycle continued, and it took me a long time to realize that I had sabotaged my own healing.

So, with 1 week left in your 21 days, really take some time to think about how you'll add foods back in starting on Day 22 and beyond. Journal where you've been, where you are now, and where you want to go, and think about what you'll have to do to get where you want to go.

NOTES

NOTES

I never wanted to live on a lake.

I grew up on gravel roads; my husband grew up on a lake in Minnesota. Together, we moved away from both to California. I've always adored the solitude of the mountains, and to me, water is not very peaceful at all. Whether it's an ocean or a lake, there is something about water that feels very overwhelming to me. Some days the water can be calm and relaxing, but then on other days it's rough, blowing, and dark, and it fills me with fear.

Yet, when it was time for our family to return to Minnesota after more than a decade away, the opportunity presented itself to purchase the home my husband had grown up in, right there on the lake. Despite my misgivings about living on the water, we decided to buy the house, and eventually I warmed up to the idea that the lake would be right outside my window. In the winters I could go down and walk on the frozen water, and in the summers, I could sit out on the dock to watch the sunshine beam off the lake.

I've lived at the lake for several seasons now, and the water is still just as changeable and unpredictable as ever. And yet there is nowhere else I'd rather be. Some days, I wake up to the reflection of the sun glistening off the water. The birds are chirping because they, too, are in their happy place. People cruise by in their boats, laughing with family and friends, getting burned to a crisp because time means nothing. But other days, I wake up and it's dark, cloudy, and raining, with thunder booming and lightning flashing.

While those days used to make me very afraid, today I embrace them. They are my reminder to slow down, stay inside, be safe, and just rest. I've learned that there is nothing to fear about the trembling or darkness or wind that sweeps over the large body of water. All I need to do on those days is stay present with them and adhere to what the lake is telling me. Slow is okay sometimes, and brighter days are ahead.

This is true, too, for your journey. As you begin the last week of this 21-day process, remember to stay present with each day. Nothing must feel too hard, dark, or overwhelming—but even if it does, you can be assured that a new day will come. Maybe the dark of your dark days is there for a reason, helping you to slow down. Instead of fighting those moments, what if you just relax into them? Stay present. If you can, sleep. Take deeper breaths. Do something that brings you joy. Just don't try so hard to get away. Fighting against the natural is never the recipe for success. Tomorrow will hopefully bring sun, but even the rain can bring its own kind of healing and growth.

CRITICAL ACTIONS TO TAKE TODAY:

☐ Get at least 8 hours of sleep.

☐ Record all bowel movements (time and type).

☐ Follow the "Say Yes" and "Say No" lists on pages 54–55 and 62–72.

☐ Choose meals from the Creations chapter on page 212.

NOTES

NOTES

- ☐ Record what you're eating—*all* the ingredients, not just the "ingredient(s)" (see page 103).
- ☐ Consume at least 8 cups of water.
- ☐ Write one line of gratitude and/or your healing mantra.
- ☐ Choose a workout activity that ranks no more than a 5 on an intensity scale of 1 to 10, and work out for a brief period of time.
- ☐ Do one thing your practitioner has told you to do but you just have not done yet.
- ☐ Record what cycle day (CD) you're on for your menstrual cycle (CD 1 = the day your period starts).

ACTIONS FOR YOU TO CONSIDER TAKING TODAY:

- ☐ Journal. Think about how you can slow down today and embrace this journey.
- ☐ Be present with your breath today. Intentionally set aside five times throughout the day to take in ten deep breaths. How do you feel afterward? Will you do this again tomorrow?

CREATION IDEAS FOR TODAY:

- ☐ Sweet Veggie Bowl (page 231)
- ☐ Beef Stroganoff Bowl (page 238)
- ☐ Breakfast Burger (page 246)

GUT REAL THOUGHT FOR TODAY:

Be miserable. Or motivate yourself. Whatever has to be done, it's always your choice. —Wayne Dyer

It's no secret I'm highly motivated by nature. Just search the terms "motivation" or "inspire" on my blog to see how often I've written about this subject. But motivation, like every other part of the Gutsy approach, is highly subjective. Wherever you are sitting today, you must dig deep to find your *own* motivation however you can. Your motivation in life, or lack thereof, will make all the difference in how you succeed with healing your gut and changing your life.

If you're *not* naturally motivated, don't let that stop you. Here are five things to try to help you find some motivation:

1. Remind yourself *why* you need to do whatever it is you're seeking to do. Figure out what's driving you, and create a vision board around that driver.
2. Set a schedule and stick to it.
3. Know when to stop and recharge. No one is motivated 24/7 and that's a fact. We all need downtime, time to recharge and refresh.
4. Dive into your effort right away. Don't wait for the ideal conditions because they may never come.
5. Celebrate every win. Celebrating even the small milestones and achievements will add fuel to your motivation and fill up your tank to help you get further on your path.

NOTES

NOTES

They say that the shortest distance between two points is a straight line. But according to scientists, "A straight line isn't always the shortest distance between two points. . . . For spherical surfaces, like Earth, great-circle distances actually represent the true shortest distance."[4]

Like a sphere, you are multidimensional. And that means your healing process will be, too. Please don't expect that you'll heal on a straight line after reading this book or completing this 21-day plan. Healing is messy, but the goal is to keep the trajectory moving in the right general direction, even if it doesn't look like a straight line.

Early on in the *A Gutsy Girl* podcast (episode 3, to be exact), I talked about thinking of healing as a circle, rather than a line.

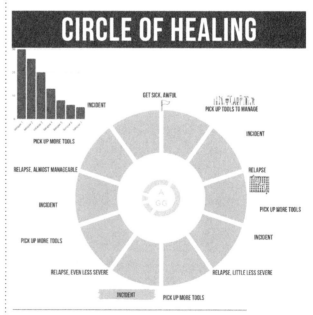

<hr />

[4]https://www.scienceabc.com/pure-sciences/is-a-straight-line-always-the-shortest-distance-between-two-points.html

In this circular model, you can see that healing is a long journey, but along the journey you'll pick up tools to help so that the next phase of healing might be easier than the one before.

And remember, the tools I need in my toolbelt may not always be the same as the tools you need in yours. Along the way, we all get to fill our toolbelts with the things we need for our own specific healing journeys. As your healing ebbs and flows, you'll figure out the perfect combination for you.

CRITICAL ACTIONS TO TAKE TODAY:

- ☐ Get at least 8 hours of sleep.
- ☐ Record all bowel movements (time and type).
- ☐ Follow the "Say Yes" and "Say No" lists on pages 54–55 and 62–72.
- ☐ Choose meals from the Creations chapter on page 212.
- ☐ Record what you're eating—*all* the ingredients, not just the "ingredient(s)" (see page 103).
- ☐ Consume at least 8 cups of water.
- ☐ Write one line of gratitude and/or your healing mantra.
- ☐ Choose a workout activity that ranks no more than a 5 on an intensity scale of 1 to 10, and work out for a brief period of time.
- ☐ Do one thing your practitioner has told you to do but you just have not done yet.
- ☐ Record what cycle day (CD) you're on for your menstrual cycle (CD 1 = the day your period starts).

NOTES

ACTIONS FOR YOU TO CONSIDER TAKING TODAY:

☐ Journal. Think about the things you currently need for your toolbelt. Are they the same as the things you needed in the past? How about things you might need for the future, but not quite yet?

☐ Try making your own Circle of Healing graphic. What does it look like? Upon completing the activity, how do you feel?

CREATION IDEAS FOR TODAY:

☐ Hempseed and Chia Bowl (page 231)

☐ Sausage and Pepper Bowl (page 239)

☐ Honey-Balsamic Chicken (page 244)

GUT REAL THOUGHT FOR TODAY:

Look back 5 years. Identify the changes already underway that you'd like to continue, reflect on any wrong turns you've made along the way, and consider the routes as yet untraveled that you'd like to explore in the future. Plan your journey and then set out with a hopeful heart.

I'm a planner. (Sometimes to a fault, as when my excessive planning takes over life!) On my healing journey, though, being a planner has served me well. I strive for better, both in the short and long term. I know where I've been. I know where I am. I know where I want to go. And all that careful planning has meant that once I set out, I never looked back. My hope is the same for you.

NOTES

When I interviewed Katie of Wellness Mama on my podcast, she said something that I think you need to hear today: "You can't heal a body you hate."

I know this can feel hard on most days. For one reason or another, many women hate the bodies they are in. And if you have any sort of chronic illness, the illness can make that feeling even worse. But I want you to go back and read the words Katie said:

You can't heal a body you hate.

So maybe it's time for you to rein those feelings of hatred in and make peace with your body, so that you *can* heal.

There are a few concrete things you can do to help with this process of making peace with your body:

Unbutton those pants. There was a time when I had far too much pride to unbutton my pants due to bloat. Refusing to unbutton them was a sort of punishment I put myself through. But the discomfort made it so much harder for me to make peace with my body. If you're feeling bloated, don't punish yourself with discomfort. Just unbutton them if you feel miserable.

Remember, sweatpants and oversized shirts are life. To this day, I wear a lot of sweatpants and sweatshirts, simply because they're comfortable. But back when my bloat was especially bad, I lived in sweats and oversized shirts. It didn't matter if it was 100 degrees outside, you would find me in sweatpants, because I felt far more confident and comfortable when I could breathe. Please don't make the mistake that many women make of worrying, "I have to look a certain way in public in order to be accepted." No one else really cares what you look like, and being comfortable is an important first step to making peace with yourself.

Journal, journal, journal. It's very important that you use your gut-healing journal to record your mental and emotional state, and how it relates to your gut, every day. By looking at the relationship between your emotions and your gut symptoms on any given day at any moment, you'll learn a lot about how powerful the mind is in the healing process. You're also likely to find patterns around your symptoms and thoughts that can help you heal.

Help others to heal yourself. I know you feel miserable, but one way to make peace with the journey, with the healing process, and with your body is by jumping outside it all for a while. Some ideas for helping others include volunteering at your church, getting involved with community activities, or helping other people who are far sicker than you are with everyday chores and by delighting them in any way possible. When I was miserable with SIBO, for example, my friend's dad had cancer. Each week I'd brew us *both* a batch of bone broth. He loved it so much that I'd receive text messages frequently from him with his unending gratitude. When we help others, we have far less time to spend focusing inward.

Remember that bloat and fat are not the same things. When you're feeling bad about the way you look, listen to your body, because deep down you know your mind has led you astray. You are not fat. Fat and bloat are not the same things. And even if they were, the bigger part of the problem is with the way you talk to yourself. If you have consistently told yourself, "Shame on you, you're fat," you have created a vicious cycle of reinforcing your own self-hatred. Break out of that damaging and stressful cycle so that you can begin to heal.

Focus on your own reflection. This is a real therapy that's recommended by professionals for various conditions. According to *Psychology Today*, "The mirror can be used to critique ourselves. But it also offers perspective on just how unkindly we're treating ourselves. Our preliminary research shows that looking with the intention to be kind to yourself can reduce anxiety and self-criticism. So, looking with kind intention can reduce anxiety, whereas looking without kind intention can allow the inner critic to run amok."[5] Practice this for yourself by standing in front of the mirror and noticing three things you like about the way you look. Focus on and embrace them.

Believe that it won't last forever. Making peace with your body while healing your gut is about so much more than any weight you may feel you have to lose. There are so many uncomfortable bodily symptoms that can coincide with gut illness: embarrassing gas, hair loss, weight gain or loss, a bloated stomach, dark circles under the eyes, acne, burping, and more, and all of them can take a toll on your ability to love yourself. One way to make peace with all of this is to know that when you heal your gut, all those other miscellaneous things will begin to heal as well. And you must believe that to find the peace you're looking for.

Do the work to heal it. This sounds simple, but it's obviously super complicated. While I do believe you need to accept your body as is while on the gut-healing journey, body

[5]https://www.psychologytoday.com/us/blog/the-clarity/201808/why-is-seeing-your-own-reflection-so-important

positivity does not mean allowing yourself to stay sick. Laughing about your symptoms to cover up your pain is not the same as making peace with your body. It's simply delaying the next inevitable mental and physical breakdown. I promise this vicious cycle will continue until you choose to prioritize your own healing.

And by the way, darling, if all else fails, know that there is a whole Gutsy community at agutsygirl .com that knows how you feel, accepts you as you are, and loves you unconditionally.

CRITICAL ACTIONS TO TAKE TODAY:

- ☐ Get at least 8 hours of sleep.
- ☐ Record all bowel movements (time and type).
- ☐ Follow the "Say Yes" and "Say No" lists on pages 54–55 and 62–72.
- ☐ Choose meals from the Creations chapter on page 212.
- ☐ Record what you're eating—*all* the ingredients, not just the "ingredient(s)" (see page 103).
- ☐ Consume at least 8 cups of water.
- ☐ Write one line of gratitude and/or your healing mantra.
- ☐ Choose a workout activity that ranks no more than a 5 on an intensity scale of 1 to 10, and work out for a brief period of time.
- ☐ Do one thing your practitioner has told you to do but you just have not done yet.
- ☐ Record what cycle day (CD) you're on for your

NOTES

menstrual cycle (CD 1 = the day your period starts).

ACTIONS FOR YOU TO CONSIDER TAKING TODAY:

☐ Journal. Try the mirror reflection activity described above and write about what you noticed and how you felt.

☐ The list above includes several ways to make peace with yourself and your body. Think about which of these you can take with you on your own journey.

CREATION IDEAS FOR TODAY:

☐ Radish Salad Bowl (page 234)

☐ Meatloaf Bowl (page 238)

☐ Spaghetti Squash with Avocado (page 248)

GUT REAL THOUGHT FOR TODAY:

Please don't ever think that you can't eat during these 21 days. The last thing I want is for Gutsy women to think that they must be hungry to succeed. Starving is not healing, because gut healing is not a diet. Here's a snippet from one of my own journals to give you an idea of how I ate during one food elimination period of my healing journey. You'll notice that there are no measurements here—I don't measure portions, and I don't use a scale. My goal is healing; nothing more, nothing less.

I was hungry from the moment I woke up at

5:30 a.m. I had a half banana and chicken with coconut oil. I worked for a few hours at the local coffee shop, so I enjoyed coffee with light coconut milk (only coconut milk, no additives or preservatives) and raw honey.

When I got home it was about 10 a.m. I was hungry so I ate a jumbo bowl of bone broth with ground kosher turkey, sprinkled with a little Himalayan pink salt and fresh-squeezed lemon juice. Still hungry after that so I had some chicken and coconut oil.

At noon I had a huge spinach salad with baby spinach, chicken, sea salt, and nutritional yeast flakes. I also had a couple raw Brazil nuts and some ground kosher turkey.

I worked out and after the workout I had a banana with my homemade Jell-O jigglers. I also had my vitamin C + l-glutamine supplements mixed in water. I drank more broth with some lemon.

When dinner rolled around, I ate another jumbo spinach salad, but this time I made it using baby spinach, smoked flank steak (Ryan homemade this last weekend—it's truly divine!) and coconut oil. And finally, for dessert I had some sea salted cinnamon almond butter.

You'll notice that I didn't eat any soda, chips,

crackers, gum, candy, or other processed food. I also didn't eat a lot of the standard "healthy" foods, like tons of vegetables or fruit, whole-grain bread, quinoa, pasta, rice, milk, or cheese. I was aware of which foods, and what quantities of those foods, my stomach dealt with well at the time, and which it did not.

There is no magic to it. There is no secret trick. I eat a ton and I move daily. I don't strive for ultimate perfection.

In due time, you'll have your routine down as well, and your gut will thrive!

There were many times on my healing journey when I became so strict and rigid with my diet that I eventually snapped. After weeks of trying to restrict and control every morsel that entered my mouth, I would snap and end up eating a whole cake or an entire tub of ice cream. Literally—I'm not even exaggerating. Afterward, I'd be miserable. And not only in the immediate aftermath or for the next few hours; I'd feel awful for days following the episode.

What I eventually learned, after healing my gut completely, is that I need to give myself an outlet for my cravings to avoid losing control completely. Today, I eat both cake and ice cream, but never to the point where I'm so stuffed that consequences follow.

And what I experienced with food is also true with emotions. I am a highly sensitive person, which means I tend to have an increased sensitivity to physical, emotional, and social stimuli. This is not a "diagnosis" or an inherently good or bad trait, but it is something that, before I was aware of it, caused me a lot of pain. Before I fully understood this trait, I never felt safe to share my sensitivity. For most of my life, I tried to restrict and control the big feelings I had, just as I had tried to excessively restrict and control my food intake. I always felt so much for my own self and on behalf of others, but those emotions stayed stuffed deep down within me. And just like with food, the pressure of constantly denying my own emotions would eventually cause me to snap.

NOTES

I did try to find an outlet for my feelings in 2008, prior to my wedding, when I saw my first therapist. I wanted to uncover what was going on, but instead of listening to what I was saying and hearing my desperation, she called afterward and left a voicemail that said, "I don't think this is going to be the right partnership."

Yes, you read that correctly. My very first therapist *fired* me.

And what happened next? You guessed it. I was afraid of seeing a new therapist for fear of being rejected again, so I just kept stuffing my emotions down, one on top of the next, and *never* dealt with any of it.

My rock bottom came years later, in October of 2018, as I shared on Day 10. At the time, I was also dealing with my dad's stage 4 colon cancer diagnosis and a rushed move back to Minnesota as well as my own illness. I finally reached the end of my emotional rope. Enough was enough and I finally went to see a doctor. After years of denying my emotions, opening up about what was happening finally allowed me to get the help I needed. I was referred to that incredible therapist and started on the medication. After years of stuffing my emotions down and arriving at dead ends when trying to unpack it all, I *finally* saw light at the end of the tunnel. Perhaps it's not surprising that this all happened shortly after I had taken my final rounds of rifaximin and neomycin, loosened the grip on my diet, and begun focusing less on working out and more on improving my overall lifestyle. To find true healing, I had to learn that emotions—like food cravings—will always find a way out. You can choose to stuff them down deeper and deeper, until one day you snap and lose control completely, or you can find a safe release valve for them. For me, in this regard, therapy was priceless.

CRITICAL ACTIONS TO TAKE TODAY:

☐ Get at least 8 hours of sleep.

☐ Record all bowel movements (time and type).

☐ Follow the "Say Yes" and "Say No" lists on pages 54–55 and 62–72.

☐ Choose meals from the Creations chapter on page 212.

☐ Record what you're eating—*all* the ingredients, not just the "ingredient(s)" (see page 103).

☐ Consume at least 8 cups of water.

☐ Write one line of gratitude and/or your healing mantra.

☐ Choose a workout activity that ranks no more than a 5 on an intensity scale of 1 to 10, and work out for a brief period of time.

☐ Do one thing your practitioner has told you to do but you just have not done yet.

☐ Record what cycle day (CD) you're on for your menstrual cycle (CD 1 = the day your period starts).

NOTES

ACTIONS FOR YOU TO CONSIDER TAKING TODAY:

☐ Journal. Where are you holding stress, anger, or sadness? Have you stuffed your emotions down instead of bringing them to the surface and addressing them?

☐ Think about something that has caused you the most emotional hardship in the past month or even decade. Have you addressed it? Why or why not?

CREATION IDEAS FOR TODAY:

☐ Fruity Loop Bowl (page 229)

☐ Saffron Chicken Bowl (page 237)

☐ Sausage Slaw Bowl (page 239)

GUT REAL THOUGHT FOR TODAY:

There are no shortcuts in life; not in business, not when it comes to our health.

This is true for a healthy lifestyle, and when it comes to *how* you heal the gut. You must be willing to hustle. Hustlin' ain't easy, and sometimes you might find yourself thinking, wouldn't it be easier to just take the shortcut? To grab the processed, prepackaged food, or the fast-food takeout? I have hustled because I care, because I'm passionate, and because I really wanted to succeed, and I've learned there truly are no short-cuts to healing. But the effort doesn't have to feel insurmountable, either. Consider that it takes no more than 10 minutes to whip up a batch of ground turkey and vegetables cooked in coconut or olive oil. If you cook five portions at once, each meal has only taken you 2 minutes to make. So who needs fast food, anyway?

Remember that stage 4 colon cancer I told you about yesterday? Well, it took my dad away from me and from the world on August 13, 2019.

On the day my dad passed, I wrote in my journal:

Today is August 13, 2019—the day Dad went to be with the Lord.

I took Georgie outside to go the bathroom late tonight. I stood in our driveway while she ran around, and I looked up at all the stars asking, "Where are you, Dad?" Tears rolled until Ryan came to hug me.

It's been close to two years since Dad was first diagnosed with cancer. He left the Earth today, on August 13, 2019, in the very early morning hours—just my mom there. He was peaceful and today I thank God that He let him go so peacefully with nothing but a few candle lights and my mom, the center and love of his life.

Today was also five weeks to the day since our lives fully turned upside down. During this time, Dad wanted us to remain private. As hard as it was, we respected his wishes. I'm glad we did because those final five weeks were really great (also hard) and super tight-knit.

I'm battling with my heart. I feel like a piece of my heart is gone, because it is. There are so many things I want to share and express, but to be honest, I don't have much logic in my mind around those thoughts. They are just there, and I am just letting them be.

I know that time will heal the awful pain that currently is, but for now, I'm just staying present with it. I'm feeling the awful hurt, but I'm also remembering all the amazing things about him. So much of who I am, for better and worse, is because of my dad. Family, good friends, his dogs, and the immaculate yard he cultivated and cared for 24/7 were his life.

I never expected to lose my dad at such a young age. And yet, I can't help but still find gratitude . . . gratitude that God gave me him as my dad and that I had 36 beautiful years knowing him. I'll continue going through photos of him. I've been calling it "hanging out with my dad." I'll put them together for his celebration of life (wake) on Friday. On Saturday, we will say our final goodbyes.

Dad told us before he left that he was in and out of another world. My mom told him, "It's a beautiful world." I must believe, no matter what, that God is there, God is here, heaven is real, and Dad is finally at peace— here with us forever.

When my dad passed away, in addition to finding a new passion for gut health and for helping those desperate to heal, I also learned the true value in meeting people where *they* are, not where I want them to be or wish they could be.

I adored my dad, yet he was as stubborn as they come. And the truth is, for years I harped on him to stop eating junk, to eat an egg or a vegetable, to stop smoking, and to see a doctor. In my defense, it all came from a place of love. But he brushed it all off. Up until the day he died, he never changed. His steadfast, stubborn constancy is one of the things I loved most about my dad, and yet it frustrated me. Why take all the Pepto, laxatives, and other masks for your gut pain, if you weren't going to change anything? I mean, it only made sense—to me, but not to him.

If I could go back in time, I wouldn't waste my time harping on my dad's diet and lifestyle. The lesson I learned is that people don't ever change because of your desire. They only change due to their own desires. And all the nagging, criticizing, shaming, blaming, and fear in the world will do nothing to change that—except maybe drive you further from the person you care about, and drive them further from the action you wish them to take.

A big part of the reason I am so passionate about gut health is because of my dad. When it comes to gut healing, we must be proactive, not reactive, and I'll never stop preaching that. But we can also only change ourselves when we are ready and willing to change.

You may be reading this right now and

wondering, "What's your point? How does this relate to me and my journey? I've never dealt with colon cancer or anything so severe."

I share my dad's story with you for two main reasons. First, it's important to know what you can and can't control. If you are Gutsy, you can only control yourself, and you cannot control everything about the way things turn out. If you are not Gutsy but are reading this to help a Gutsy loved one, know that you *must* let go of your desires for them—just love them unconditionally, because that's what they need.

Finally, I share this story with you because my dad was constantly told, "It's just IBS."

Darling, it's *never* "just IBS." Promise me you'll never settle there.

CRITICAL ACTIONS TO TAKE TODAY:

- [ ] Get at least 8 hours of sleep.
- [ ] Record all bowel movements (time and type).
- [ ] Follow the "Say Yes" and "Say No" lists on pages 54–55 and 62–72.
- [ ] Choose meals from the Creations chapter on page 212.
- [ ] Record what you're eating—*all* the ingredients, not just the "ingredient(s)" (see page 103).
- [ ] Consume at least 8 cups of water.
- [ ] Write one line of gratitude and/or your healing mantra.
- [ ] Choose a workout activity that ranks no more than a 5 on an intensity scale of 1 to 10, and work out for a brief period of time.

☐ Do one thing your practitioner has told you to do but you just have not done yet.

☐ Record what cycle day (CD) you're on for your menstrual cycle (CD 1 = the day your period starts).

ACTIONS FOR YOU TO CONSIDER TAKING TODAY:

☐ Journal. Today just write about letting go. Write about letting something or someone go. I know, I know—it's not easy. Not at all. But like my journal entry the day my dad passed helped me to process the moment, writing about your own losses can be a huge help in processing where you are on your journey.

☐ Is there someone in your life who you just need to accept instead of trying to change them? Write about the person and what you'll accept about them.

CREATION IDEAS FOR TODAY:

☐ Cauliflower Bowl (page 235)
☐ Pork Bowl (page 238)
☐ Slightly Sweet Burger (page 246)

GUT REAL THOUGHT FOR TODAY:

You will get lost, but you will never accept getting lost as your final destination.

Lest you think I lead a 100% perfectly Gutsy lifestyle, I do *not*. I am just like you: I have setbacks, and you must expect that you will, too. None of us live in a bubble (though I sometimes wish I could!). Typically, a setback doesn't happen because of one day or one meal; it happens because life happens, and in times of stress, it can be easy to get off track.

When you have a setback, the first thing to do is to *recognize* you've been set back. And then, it's time for a reset. For me, this means cutting everything, cold turkey, and getting back to basics. If you've been stringent about following this 21-day plan up to now, you know what this feels like. There is no "kind of–sort of" in getting yourself back on track—you need to turn to your tried and tested, trusted courses of action. If you settle for mediocrity, you'll never find your way back to the right path again. Don't settle for lost as your destination. You *know* what to do. You *know* where you want to go. You *know* the correct path to healing.

NOTES

NOTES

Heal your gut. Heal your life: **It's my mantra, my tagline, and my motto for the entire Gutsy community.** My story may have different patterns and themes from yours, but there's one thing we all have in common: during this Gutsy journey, we are not our best selves. I don't mean you need to strive to be anything but exactly who you are; what I'm talking about are the negative thoughts and voices that fill your minds and days. I'm talking about the way your misery doesn't just seep throughout your entire body, but also pours onto the people around you, and maybe even drenches those you love most.

When you heal your gut, though, you heal your life—all the parts of your life. It's a ripple effect that happens. Your healing starts within and then extends beyond you to affect every single person you touch in the world.

Remember, 70 to 80% of your immune system cells can be found in the gut, and it is estimated that the gut produces 90% of the body's serotonin as well.[6] Your gut is your nucleus; your health and happiness both literally and figuratively have deep roots there. When your gut heals, your life—every last thing about it—also has the chance to heal.

The beautiful thing is that the reverse is also true: healing your life will also help you begin to heal your gut. This all starts with you, and the only way things can begin to improve is if you change

---

[6]https://journals.physiology.org/doi/full/10.1152/ajpgi.1999.277.5.g922

the thing that truly needs changing. The thing that needs to change is not your constipation, bloating, or diarrhea. Those are just the symptoms and manifestations of whatever it is that does need to change. For you, perhaps the thing that truly needs changing is your mindset, diet, sleep schedule, water consumption, or stress management.

Healing your gut and your life can be a long and complicated journey, but it's critical that you never stop striving to reach that destination. Be honest with yourself—when you heal your gut, how will that change your life? How will it change the lives of those you love, and how will it change the world around you?

I was once in your shoes, and I'm here to tell you that on the other side, everything changes for the better. Start today by writing it down as today's mantra, and really embracing it: *Heal your gut. Heal your life.*

CRITICAL ACTIONS TO TAKE TODAY:

- ☐ Get at least 8 hours of sleep.
- ☐ Record all bowel movements (time and type).
- ☐ Follow the "Say Yes" and "Say No" lists on pages 54–55 and 62–72.
- ☐ Choose meals from the Creations chapter on page 212.
- ☐ Record what you're eating—*all* the ingredients, not just the "ingredient(s)" (see page 103).
- ☐ Consume at least 8 cups of water.

NOTES

☐ Write one line of gratitude and/or your healing mantra.

☐ Choose a workout activity that ranks no more than a 5 on an intensity scale of 1 to 10, and work out for a brief period of time.

☐ Do one thing your practitioner has told you to do but you just have not done yet.

☐ Record what cycle day (CD) you're on for your menstrual cycle (CD 1 = the day your period starts).

ACTIONS FOR YOU TO CONSIDER TAKING TODAY:

☐ Journal. Try to finish this sentence: "When I heal my gut and heal my life, then. . . ."

☐ What do you think are the things that need changing in your life? Remember, it's *not* your bowel movements, bloat, and/or constipation. Those are just the results.

CREATION IDEAS FOR TODAY:

☐ Squash Breakfast Bowl (page 230)

☐ Italian Bowl (page 238)

☐ Tropical Smoothie (page 221)

GUT REAL THOUGHT FOR TODAY:

I have not failed. I've just found 10,000 ways that won't work. —Thomas A. Edison

It's true. You have *not* failed. Until now, perhaps the things you have tried simply haven't worked. Or maybe they did work, but they were done in combination with something else that wasn't working. On my decade-plus-long journey toward healing my gut, I definitely tried thousands of things that didn't work. And sometimes the issue wasn't that they didn't work, but that the sum of the parts at any given time wasn't working on my behalf. There is no failure, though, if you never give up.

NOTES

Today is the last day of your 21-day journey, and I want to leave you today with the six words that have guided my life since early in my own journey.

Everything is beautiful in its time.

This phrase comes from the Bible, Ecclesiastes 3:11. I believe so strongly in these six words that I turned them into a tattoo—III:XI—etched on my inner right wrist.

I first heard this passage in my twenties, when I started going to a young women's Bible study group. The women in the group shared a lot of personal stuff, but each week I stayed quiet. Maybe it was because I didn't know these women very well, or just because, as I mentioned previously, I was programmed to keep things very tight to the vest and not show my own emotion. But week after week, I'd listen as the others shared stories of infidelity, assault, abuse, and more, and feeling like my circumstances were less than, would stay silent

Then, one week, the conversation turned toward the subject of things we had been longing for. As we went around the circle, I was dreading my time to speak up, telling myself to keep it together, because the thing I had been longing for was very clear and obvious: a baby. When my turn arrived, it all poured out. I cried as I spoke of our desire to have a baby, and how month after month, it was not happening.

After I shared, a very young woman spoke up and said, "I have something I want to share with you from the Bible." This woman was probably the person in the group who I felt the least connection with, and in that moment, I assumed there was nothing she could possibly have to offer that would connect with how I was feeling, how I had been feeling for months on end.

Then she read, "Everything is beautiful in its time."

She promised that eventually, I would see what the words meant, and their message would become very clear. When I left that night, I felt a different connection to the Bible than I ever had before. Those six words never left my mind or my heart, and now, years later, everything in my life is exemplified by this phrase. I never gave birth to children, but instead was blessed with three beautiful babies we adopted from the foster care system in California. I cannot imagine a life without them. Even the way I healed, and the timing of my healing just before my dad passed, was something I could never have predicted. Yet it's meant more to me than it would have had I healed years earlier.

I think about the children, my dad, healing my gut, my relationships, living arrangement, career—all of it. Somehow everything has been beautiful, but only in its time.

Whether or not you are religious, I believe these words have value for all of us. My hope is that someday you, too, will look back and say, "Wow, how true it is that everything is beautiful in its own time."

You don't have to love every moment of your gut-healing journey—in fact, you won't, and that's

NOTES

completely normal. But to heal and get better, you do have to remember what I said on day one: *Nothing changes if nothing changes.* The journey is long, and there may be moments where you can't see where you're headed or why. Just remember, everything is beautiful in its own time. And darling, it's your time!

CRITICAL ACTIONS TO TAKE TODAY:

☐ Get at least 8 hours of sleep.

☐ Record all bowel movements (time and type).

☐ Follow the "Say Yes" and "Say No" lists on pages 54–55 and 62–72.

☐ Choose meals from the Creations chapter on page 212.

☐ Record what you're eating—*all* the ingredients, not just the "ingredient(s)" (see page 103).

☐ Consume at least 8 cups of water.

☐ Write one line of gratitude and/or your healing mantra.

☐ Choose a workout activity that ranks no more than a 5 on an intensity scale of 1 to 10, and work out for a brief period of time.

☐ Do one thing your practitioner has told you to do but you just have not done yet.

☐ Record what cycle day (CD) you're on for your menstrual cycle (CD 1 = the day your period starts).

ACTIONS FOR YOU TO CONSIDER TAKING TODAY:

☐ Journal. If you look back, can you think of a time in your past when you can say everything happened at the right time, as it should have?

☐ Do the critical actions for today, and then make your *own* list of critical actions to take in the next 3 days. Are they the same as what you've been doing for the past 21 days? Or are there new things you want to focus on based on what you know about yourself today, on Day 21?

CREATION IDEAS FOR TODAY:

☐ Thankful Bowl (page 236)
☐ Papaya Bowl (page 231)
☐ Marinated Eggs (page 248)

GUT REAL THOUGHT FOR TODAY:

A habit is first cobwebs, then cables.
—North American proverb

Creating new habits can be messy in the beginning because old habits die hard. If you don't allow those bad habits to die hard, you'll never make the necessary connections to build new, healthier habits. For the past 21 days, you've been working hard to break all the habits that have been holding you back from healing. As you move forward and your freshly created "good" habits form, you'll be confident that they are forming the cables you need for continued gut health.

NOTES

You've made it through the 21 days—so what's next? Here are three things to keep in mind as you look forward:

1. Healing your gut is *far more* than a 21-day journey. Please remember that it's an entire commitment. I hope these 21 days have given you the inspiration to keep going and to keep seeking answers.

2. If you're feeling good after these 21 days, perhaps your body just needed a reset. In that case, be sure to start incorporating more foods back into your daily life.

3. The Gutsy community is always here for you! Join us online at agutsygirl.com, on Instagram (@agutsygirl), via YouTube (*A Gutsy Girl*), and on the *A Gutsy Girl* podcast.

NOTES

A GUTSY GIRL'S
CREATIONS

As diet is one of the three main pillars to ultimate healing, this bible would not be complete without a food component. This section is intended to help you start off on the right track and make the right dietary changes for your gut-healing journey.

If there is one thing I've learned about diet on my journey, it is that no one diet or plan works for everyone. This is why I've decided to offer you what I call "Creations," rather than traditional recipes. When we can do things our own way, based on our own circumstances, we feel far less restricted and more empowered to make positive changes.

Many of the Creations in this book hardly give any instruction. This is intentional. My goal was to identify healing and nutritious ingredients that, when combined, taste great together. However, for one reason or another, different people tolerate food quantities, cooking methods, and ingredient combinations differently. Therefore, the Creations allow you to do what works best for you. I encourage you to use my basic formulas as a jumping-off point to get inspired and come up with your own Creations. One hundred percent personalization is the key to healing and compliance.

Ingredients

All Creations that follow use ingredients from the "Say Yes" list on page 54, making them safe choices for your 21-day journey. However, you can also swap in your own favorite ingredients for any of these Creations, if you're careful to stick with safe choices you know will work for your own body.

Essential Equipment for the Gutsy Girl's Kitchen

Healing your gut requires cooking at home, and before you can get started, you'll need to have the right tools. In addition to the basic kitchen tools, there are a few items that can make it easier to cook and eat specifically for gut health. Here are my top recommendations for stocking your Gutsy Girl kitchen:

Cheesecloth: I use cheesecloth mostly for making my own nondairy milk, but it can also be used to make other drinks and smooth sauces. I even use it sometimes to make fresh juices—just puree your fruit or veggies in a blender and then strain through cheesecloth for the same effect you'd get with a juicer. You can find inexpensive packages of cheesecloth at the dollar store.

Looking for nutritional information for each Creation? You won't find it in *A Gutsy Girl's Bible*. The reason is very simple. Healing the gut is not about counting calories. Instead, it's about counting ingredients and paying attention to the foods and ingredients that work for you on your specific journey. The more we focus on counting calories and worrying about a number on the scale, the less we are able to focus on what really matters—healing.

Food Processor: I make everything from soups to sauces, fudge to casseroles and more in my food processor. The sky is the limit and making these items from scratch with a food processor is far more beneficial to your gut-healing journey than using the packaged versions. I have a Cuisinart 14-cup food processor, and I recommend you don't go any smaller than that.

GarlicZoom: Love garlic, but hate chopping it up all the time? Enter the GarlicZoom. Simply place your (peeled) garlic in and roll (aka "zoom"). It has saved me so much time! I also use mine to mince ginger.

Hand Blender: A hand blender makes it super simple to create soups, sauces, puddings, and even homemade applesauce. I use the Cuisinart Hand Blender. It's easy to use and clean, and so small that it can be stored in even the tiniest kitchen.

Handheld Drink Mixer/Milk Frother: My Nestpark Portable Drink Mixer is the best $15 I've ever spent on a kitchen tool. This is a must if you like making gut-healing lattes or blending MCT oil and other "bulletproof oils" into your coffee. The portable style means you can take it on the go with you or use it in the comfort of your own home; either way, you'll get the frothiness you want without the need for any large, expensive equipment.

High-Speed Blender: I use my Vitamix for almost everything—smoothies, dressings, desserts, sauces, and more! As I mentioned above, juices are better than smoothies when you're first starting out on your healing journey. But ultimately your gut should heal to a place where you can consume all the fiber a smoothie contains.

Instant Pot: The incredible Instant Pot allows you to make everything from broths to beverages to hard-boiled eggs in a hurry, saving you precious time. One of my favorite things to do with the Instant Pot is make vegetable broth and bone broth.

Juicer: If you are a Gutsy Girl, having a fresh juice is *not* the same as having a smoothie. While a regular blender will not remove the skins and other roughage from your fruits and veggies, the juicer will. Juicing allows you to get all the nutrients out of your produce, with none of the misery.

Lemon Squeezer: Lemon is a great addition to so many dishes. I use lemon juice in my daily doses of broth, and the lemon squeezer makes the process simple and clean.

Muffin Pan: Muffin pans aren't just for muffins anymore! I use my regular- and mini muffin pans for portion control with baked dishes, snacks, and more! One of my favorite recipes to make in my muffin pan is turkey meatloaf muffins.

Personal-Size Blender: A mini blender allows you to make smaller portions of blended items with less mess and cleanup. I use the Nutri Ninja Pro, and I love how small the containers are, and the fact that you can take it on the go, if need be.

Slow Cooker: Slow and go is a great gut-healing, cooking, and general life motto. I have a Calphalon 7-quart Digital Slow Cooker, which I use to make meat dishes and bone broths primarily.

Spiralizer: The spiralizer will change your foodie life. I use mine mostly to spiralize zucchini noodles, but there are a whole host of foods that can be successfully spiralized. Spiralizing vegetables is a great way to add fiber to your diet while reducing wheat and gluten, which is typically critical in any 21-day program.

Steamer: Steaming your vegetables will make them softer and easier to digest. You can get a stand-alone steamer or purchase one that comes paired with other items. For example, I have a rice cooker that includes a steamer basket that can be set on top.

Wok: My wok is one of my favorite tools for large-batch cooking. I like to create huge stir-fry meals and then divide them up to conquer eating healthy throughout the week. Remember, batch cooking is an easy way to enjoy "fast food" later in the week.

JUICES

To correctly make a juice, you need to have a juicer. Simply run all the ingredients through your juicer; no peeling or seeding necessary. If you do not have a juicer, you can still make juice but it's just more time consuming. To make juice sans juicer, combine all the ingredients together in a blender and then strain the juice through a piece of cheesecloth to remove any remaining solids. Each of the Creations in this section will make one to two servings.

Juice all ingredients in a juicer and serve immediately.

NOTES

APPLE-KALE JUICE

1 apple

1 beet

A few handfuls kale

Ground cinnamon, for sprinkling

CUCUMBER-APPLE-MINT JUICE

1 cucumber

1 apple

A few fresh mint leaves

Several handfuls kale and/or spinach

1 cup chopped pineapple

ENERGIZING JUICE

1 cucumber

3 celery stalks

Several handfuls kale and/or spinach

A few fresh mint leaves

¼ lemon (with peel, if desired and organic)

1 orange

FRUITY AND LIGHT JUICE

2 kiwifruit

1 apple

1 cucumber

3 celery stalks

Almond or coconut milk, for topping (optional)

PURPLE JUICE

1 cup blueberries

Several handfuls purple kale

2 large carrots

2 celery stalks

1 peach

1 cucumber

1 small lemon

JUST GREEN JUICE

1 green apple

1 cucumber

½ lemon

3 celery stalks

1 small slice ginger (optional)

NO-FRUIT JUICE

Several handfuls spinach

1 cup broccoli

3 celery stalks

3 carrots

Almond or coconut milk, for topping (optional)

TO THE "BEET" JUICE

1 apple

2 celery stalks

3 carrots

Almond or coconut milk, for topping (optional)

WAKE-UP JUICE

1 cup broccoli

3 carrots

1 apple

2 celery stalks

1 small lemon

ALKALINE LOVE JUICE

3 celery stalks

1 cucumber

3 carrots

1 green apple

Several handfuls spinach

SMOOTHIES

Remember, the point of a smoothie is to include the skin for extra fiber and nutrition, but this isn't going to work for everyone at all times. Pay attention to how you feel after drinking a smoothie versus drinking a juice. If you find that at certain points on your journey, the added fiber is not working for you, stick to juices instead. The Creations below will each make one to two smoothies.

Combine all ingredients in a blender; blend and serve.

BERRIES 'N' GREENS SMOOTHIE

1 cup almond milk

1 cup frozen berries of choice

3 large handfuls kale and/or spinach

COCONUTTY SMOOTHIE

1 cup coconut milk

3 large handfuls greens of choice

½ tablespoon coconut oil

1 cup frozen fruit of choice

2 tablespoons unsweetened shredded coconut

BERRY-LICIOUS HEMP SMOOTHIE

1 banana, fresh or frozen (about 1 cup)

2 tablespoons organic hempseed

½ cup blueberries, fresh or frozen

½ cup raspberries, fresh or frozen

½ cup milk of choice

2 teaspoons vanilla extract

½ tablespoon fresh mint leaves

2 heaping handfuls fresh spinach

10 ice cubes

NOTES

SPA WATERS

Do you have a hard time drinking water because it tastes "too bland"? Make spa water instead—simply add fresh herbs, fruits, and other ingredients to plain water to naturally flavor your water. I've listed 18 flavor combinations here to get you started, but you can think creatively and use any other fruits, vegetables, or herbs you like. Whatever flavors you choose, be sure to use fresh, whole foods, such as fresh mint or thyme and freshly sliced peaches, pears, or cucumbers.

Cucumber + mint

Watermelon + mint

Cucumber + basil

Pear + lime + ginger

Peach + basil

Orange + mint

Apple + fennel

Lemon + thyme

Orange + rosemary + fennel

Strawberry + mint

Raspberry + basil

Blackberry + mint

Lemon + ginger

Strawberry + cucumber

Cherry + thyme

Pineapple + mint + ginger

Orange + thyme

Peach + lavender

MINT-LIME 'NANA SHAKE

1 green apple, cored and quartered

½ small lime, peeled

2 cups frozen chopped bananas

½ cup full-fat coconut milk

½ cup coconut milk light

1 tablespoon fresh mint

½ cup ice cubes

TROPICAL SMOOTHIE

½ cup frozen pineapple

½ frozen chopped banana

1 cup coconut milk

1 tablespoon unsweetened, shredded coconut

CREAMY COCONUT-BANANA MINT SHAKE

1 or 2 frozen chopped bananas

½ to 1 cup coconut milk

1 tablespoon fresh mint leaves

ice cubes

OTHER BEVERAGES

Beverages are single serve. They can be doubled for another person or to save for a different time. Fruit infusions can be for however many people you want to serve or throughout the day replenished with water. Fruit drinks will taste the best consumed on the same day.

Combine all ingredients and stir. Serve lemonade over ice. Serve the coffee and hot cocoa hot.

NOTES

GINGER LEMONADE

1 cup freshly squeezed lemon juice

¼ cup peeled fresh ginger slices

7 sprigs mint

2 cups water

BANANA COFFEE

1 medium banana

½ cup milk of choice

8 to 12 ounces coffee

HOT COCOA

2 tablespoons unsweetened cocoa powder

1 cup milk of choice, heated

1 tablespoon maple syrup or honey

HOMEMADE COFFEE CREAMERS

Make a large batch of gut-friendly homemade coffee creamer and store in the freezer so it's always ready when you need it! Mix and match the different flavor options as you please within each batch (I use a dry-erase marker to label the molds, so I don't forget which flavor is which).

Whisk the coconut milk by hand for 2 to 3 minutes and then pour into individual candy molds. Add your desired flavoring(s) to each mold and freeze. Use as needed to flavor your coffee.

1 can full-fat coconut milk, refrigerated overnight

FLAVORING OPTIONS:

Coconut sugar

100% cacao powder

Honey

Ground cinnamon

Almond extract

Coffee extract

Peppermint extract

Orange extract

Vanilla extract

Coconut extract

NOTES

DRESSINGS AND SAUCES

Dressings and sauces were the spice to my gut-healing life! Honestly, having the ability to pour dressings and sauces over salads, meats, steamed or roasted vegetables, and so on makes it so much easier to comply with a strict diet. Whenever you need a burst of flavor, head to the dressings and sauces Creations. Each of the Creations below makes enough for one serving or more, depending on how you plan to use it. Whatever you do not use can be stored for up to a week.

Vinaigrettes

Combine all ingredients in a jar with a lid and shake vigorously.

NOTES

GARLIC-SAGE VINAIGRETTE

½ cup garlic-infused coconut oil

2 tablespoons lemon juice

1 tablespoon + 1 teaspoon maple syrup

1 teaspoon finely chopped fresh sage

½ teaspoon ground cinnamon

¼ teaspoon salt

SIMPLE VINAIGRETTE

3 tablespoons olive oil

1 tablespoon apple cider vinegar

Pinch of sea salt

Pinch of ground cinnamon

LIQUID COCONUT OIL VINAIGRETTE

½ cup liquid coconut oil

¼ cup apple cider vinegar

2 tablespoons coconut aminos

1 sprig rosemary

MAPLE GARLIC DRESSING

½ cup garlic-infused coconut oil

1 tablespoon maple syrup

3 tablespoons apple cider vinegar

½ tablespoon chopped fresh thyme

Salt to taste

SIMPLE HERBED VINEGAR

While I've used tarragon here as an example, this basic vinegar can be made with any of your favorite fresh herbs.

BASIC TARRAGON VINEGAR

¼ to ½ cup white vinegar

Few sprigs fresh tarragon

Combine ingredients in a jar; cover and let sit for 5 to 7 days before enjoying.

BLENDED DRESSINGS AND SAUCES

Dressing and sauces can be made on a meal prep day or when you have the ingredients on hand. You can use them all week on multiple bowls and dishes. Use the amount you desire according to your taste. Sauces can spruce up any meal and be a nice addition to many dishes.

Combine all ingredients in a small blender. Blend until completely mixed and smooth.

NOTES

CITRUS DRESSING

Juice of 1 lemon

¼ cup oil

1 garlic clove, roasted

2 tablespoons fresh herbs of choice

CREAMY DRESSING

1 (8- to 10-oz.) can coconut milk

¼ cup fresh herbs of choice

2 tablespoons citrus juice or apple cider vinegar

1 shallot

HOMEMADE BLUEBERRY VINAIGRETTE

¼ cup blueberries

2 tablespoons white balsamic vinegar

½ tablespoon olive oil

Pinch of sea salt

AVOCADO SAUCE

1 avocado

Juice of 1 lime or lemon

1 clove garlic

¼ cup coconut milk

ITALIAN SAUCE

1 (28-ounce) can diced tomatoes or 4 cups fresh diced tomatoes

¼ cup fresh basil

3 tablespoons oil

2 garlic cloves

1 small onion, finely chopped

NON-DAIRY TZATZIKI SAUCE

1½ cups full-fat coconut milk, chilled in the fridge overnight

1 cup peeled, seeded, diced cucumber

Juice of ½ lemon

1 tablespoon chopped fresh dill

2 garlic cloves, peeled

¼ teaspoon sea salt

¼ teaspoon pepper

BOWLS

Bowls are a simple way to put different flavors, textures, and nutrients together to keep things fresh, simple, and delicious. For all bowls, simply prepare the ingredients ahead of time (for example, cook bacon, bake sweet potatoes, and slice or chop veggies) and then build your bowl however you desire. The portions and amounts per ingredient indicated below will generally feed two to four people. Whatever you don't eat can be saved for later so you can cook once and enjoy several meals throughout the week (on-the-go healing at its finest!). Remember, there is no right way to do any of it. The only "right way" is the way that works for you. Want whole strips of bacon vs. chopped, then create your bowl that way. Prefer sliced fruit over diced? Go for it!

Prepare all ingredients as desired; then layer in a bowl.

Breakfast

NOTES

BACON BOWL

1 pound cooked bacon

3 bananas

¼ cup chia seeds

3 medium sweet potatoes

1 cup almond milk

Maple syrup, for drizzling

BREAKFAST FRUIT BOWL

2 cups melon

2 bananas

2 cups coconut milk

1 cup blueberries

½ cup almonds

Ground cinnamon, for garnish

Hempseed or chia seeds, for garnish

NUTTY BOWL

2 cup walnuts

1 cup berries of choice

2 bananas

½ cup nut butter of choice

2 tablespoons honey

Ground cinnamon, for garnish

Hempseed or chia seeds, for garnish

PACKED PROTEIN BOWL

1 package chicken sausage, cooked

1 pound cooked bacon

2 tablespoons freshly chopped sage, tarragon, or rosemary

1 large onion

1 small/medium bag Brussels sprouts

Maple syrup or honey, for drizzling

PAPAYA SUNRISE BOWL

1 papaya

¼ cup unsweetened shredded coconut

½ cup blueberries

2 tablespoons chia seeds or hempseed

¼ cup nut butter of choice

Ground cinnamon, for sprinkling

FRUITY LOOPY BOWL

1 cup raspberries

1 cup strawberries

FRUITY LOOPY BOWL (continued)

1 cup blueberries

Milk of choice (enough to cover the berries)

½ cup walnuts

Cacao nibs, chia seeds, hempseed, or hazelnuts, for garnish

SPRINGTIME PROTEIN BOWL

2 cups cooked turkey or chicken sausage

1 bunch asparagus

2 shallots

8 ounces mushrooms

¼ cup fresh parsley

SQUASH BREAKFAST BOWL

1 winter squash or 1 small bag frozen squash

2 bananas

1 pound cooked bacon

1 onion

Maple syrup, for drizzling

Walnuts, for garnish

SIMPLE SALAD MORNING BOWL

2 cups arugula or spinach

1 apple

1 pound cooked bacon

¼ cup fresh parsley

Lemon juice, honey, and oil, for drizzling

Optional: scrambled eggs

FRUIT BOWL

4 bananas

2 cups blueberries

¼ cup unsweetened shredded coconut

1 can coconut milk

Ground cinnamon, for garnish

Nuts of choice, for garnish

PAPAYA BOWL

1 papaya

½ cup blueberries

¼ cup unsweetened shredded coconut

2 tablespoons chia seeds

Nuts of choice

HEMPSEED AND CHIA BOWL

¼ cup hempseed

¼ cup chia seeds

1 cup nut or seed milk of choice

Berries of choice, for garnish

Ground cinnamon, for garnish

Salad and Veggie Bowls

SWEET VEGGIE BOWL

4 medium sweet potatoes

½ cup nut butter

1 tablespoon chia seeds

1 teaspoon ground cinnamon

1 apple, diced

CUCUMBER BOWL

2 cucumbers

2 tablespoons mint

2 tablespoons pepitas

recipe continued on page 234

BUILD-YOUR-OWN PALEO SMOOTHIE BOWL

You can build your *own* smoothie bowl to fit whatever your cravings are or your diet necessities might be. To make this bowl, simply choose a base ingredient, blend with whatever other items you want to add to it, and serve in a bowl with your preferred toppings. My experience is that the best smoothie bowls start with a semi-frozen base. So, for instance, if you want a banana base, freeze your bananas prior to blending them. If this is a smoothie bowl built for one, use ½ to 1 cup fruit for your base (e.g., 1 cup frozen banana).

BASE INGREDIENTS:

Banana	Pear	Strawberries
Apple	Kiwifruit	Blueberries
Orange	Avocado	Raspberries
Mango	Cherry	Blackberries
Peach	Pineapple	

GREEN ADD-INS:

Kale

Spinach

Chard

LIQUID ADD-INS:

Coconut water

100% fruit juice

Nondairy milk (coconut, almond, cashew, walnut, hemp, etc.)

PROTEIN ADD-INS:

Protein powder

Coconut milk yogurt

ADD-INS FOR NUTRIENTS, COLOR, TEXTURE, AND FLAVOR:

Chia seeds	Honey	Maple syrup
Hempseed	Cinnamon	Matcha powder
Flaxseed	Turmeric	Vanilla
Almonds	Ginger	Spirulina
Coconut manna	Maca	
Coconut oil	Peanut butter	

CRUNCHY TOPPINGS:

Chia seeds	Pumpkin seeds	Pomegranate seeds
Hempseed	Walnuts	Cacao nibs
Sunflower seeds	Almonds	

OTHER TOPPINGS:

Banana	Strawberries	Dried fruit
Mango	Blueberries	Coconut whipped cream
Peach	Raspberries	Bee pollen
Pear	Blackberries	
Kiwifruit	Dragon fruit	
Pineapple	Unsweetened shredded coconut	

NOTES

CUCUMBER BOWL (continued)

¼ cup parsley

Juice of 1 lime

BLACKBERRY SALAD BOWL

⅔ cup blackberries

2 cups cooked chicken

¼ cup purple onion

1 avocado

¼ cup walnuts

Optional: lettuce mixture of choice

EGG ROLL SALAD BOWL

1 pound cooked protein of choice

4 cups cooked cabbage

½ cup scallions

½ cup carrots

¼ cup cashews or sunflower seeds

Optional: lettuce mixture of choice

RADISH SALAD BOWL

1 cucumber

1 radish

1 lemon

¼ cup fresh dill

3 tablespoons olive oil

SALAD BOWL

4 cups greens of choice

1 pound cooked protein of choice (about 2 cups)

½ cup radishes

½ cup olives

Nuts of choice, for garnish

Fresh herbs of choice, for garnish

Dressing of choice, for drizzling

CAULIFLOWER BOWL

1 head cauliflower, riced or 1 bag frozen riced cauliflower

¼ cup fresh parsley or 2 tablespoons dried

¼ cup pistachios

1 pound cooked protein of choice

SQUASH BOWL

1 spaghetti squash

1 cup tomatoes

1 pound cooked protein of choice

¼ cup fresh parsley

1 cup spinach

Protein Bowls

BEACH BOWL

4 cooked cod fillets

¼ cup unsweetened shredded coconut

1 small onion, thinly sliced

4 cups sliced cabbage or 1 bag coleslaw mix

Fresh cilantro, for garnish

Citrus wedges, for garnish

SALMON BOWL

3 cooked salmon fillets

¾ cup cucumber

2 teaspoons freshly grated ginger

SALMON BOWL (continued)

1 avocado

4 cups greens

Citrus wedges and/or zest, for garnish

Sesame seeds, for garnish

WILD SALMON AND HEMPSEED CAULIFLOWER RICE BOWL

4 to 6 ounces cooked wild salmon

1 head cauliflower, riced, or 1 bag frozen riced cauliflower

2 tablespoons hempseed oil

1 tablespoon hempseed, or as desired

Sea salt, to taste

THANKFUL BOWL

1 pound cooked ground turkey or 2 cups diced turkey

4 cups squash or sweet potatoes

1 large onion

4 celery stalks

Chopped apples, for garnish

Nuts of choice, for garnish

HARVEST BOWL

2 cups cooked chicken or 1 pound cooked ground chicken

4 cups arugula

1 cup cherries

2 cups sweet potatoes

Nuts of choice, for garnish

Dressing of choice, for drizzling

SAFFRON CHICKEN BOWL

1 to 1½ pounds cooked chicken

Pinch of saffron

1 medium onion

1 (16-ounce) can tomatoes

3 garlic cloves

CHICKEN AND SQUASH BOWL

1 pound cooked ground chicken

3 yellow squash

10 ounces cherry tomatoes

¼ cup fresh basil

Salt and pepper to taste

Balsamic vinegar, for drizzling

DUCK BOWL

2 cups cooked duck

½ cup cherries, dried or fresh

2 to 3 medium sweet potatoes

Dash of ground cinnamon

BEEF BOWL

1 pound cooked beef sirloin or ground beef

2 bunches bok choy

4 cups Brussels sprouts

¼ cup fresh basil

¼ cup fresh cilantro

Coconut aminos and lime juice, for drizzling

ROAST BEEF BOWL

2 cups cooked sliced roast beef

¼ cup fresh dill or 2 tablespoons dried

ROAST BEEF BOWL (continued)

1 bag green beans

3 large carrots

BEEF STROGANOFF BOWL

1 to 1½ pounds cooked beef

8 ounces mushrooms

1 onion

½ cup coconut milk

2 garlic cloves

Optional: spiralized vegetable of choice (zucchini, squash, etc.)

MEATLOAF BOWL

1 pound cooked ground beef

1 red bell pepper

1 onion

3 tablespoons tomato paste

Green beans or other vegetable of choice, for serving

PORK BOWL

1 pound cooked ground pork or 2 cups diced pork

4 cups Brussels sprouts

4 cups squash or sweet potatoes

¼ cups chives

½ cup apples

Creamy dressing, for drizzling

ITALIAN BOWL

1 pound cooked meat of choice

2 zucchini

1 bunch or 1 medium bag of broccoli

8 ounces mushrooms

Italian Sauce (page 227), for topping

CHILI BOWL

1 pound cooked ground meat of choice

½ pound bacon

1 onion

1 (28-ounce) can tomatoes

1 tablespoon chili powder

Avocado, for garish

Fresh cilantro, for garnish

LAMB BOWL

1 pound cooked lamb

¼ cup fresh mint

¼ cup pistachios

Juice of 1 lemon

2 pounds green beans

SAUSAGE SLAW BOWL

1 pound cooked sausage of choice

1 small bag of cabbage slaw mix

¼ cup fresh cilantro

¼ cup sunflower seeds

Honey and vinegar, for drizzling

SAUSAGE AND PEPPER BOWL

1 pound cooked sausage

2 bell peppers of choice

2 portobello mushrooms

¼ cup tomato paste

Cooked cauliflower rice, for serving

Fresh basil, for garnish

BROTHS AND SOUP BOWLS

There are two main ways I make broths: Instant Pot and stove top.

Broths

NOTES

BEEF BONE BROTH

1 pound beef bones

2 tablespoons olive oil

Salt

Freshly ground black pepper

3 bay leaves

2 garlic cloves, unpeeled, chopped

2 carrots, unpeeled, cut into thirds (plus carrot tops, if you have them)

1 celery stalk, cut into thirds

½ leek, cut into thirds

½ red onion, unpeeled, chopped

½ yellow onion, unpeeled, chopped

½ bunch fresh flat-leaf parsley, chopped

2 tablespoons apple cider vinegar

CHICKEN BONE BROTH

1 pound chicken bones (plus any leftover giblets from cooking whole chicken, if you have them)

2 carrots, unpeeled, cut into thirds (plus carrot tops, if you have them)

2 garlic cloves, unpeeled, chopped

2 bay leaves

1 celery stalk, cut into thirds

1 lemon, halved

½ leek, cut into thirds

½ red onion, unpeeled, cut into thirds

½ yellow onion, unpeeled, cut into thirds

small handful fresh rosemary

½ bunch fresh cilantro, chopped

15 cups water

2 tablespoons apple cider vinegar

½ (¾-ounce) package fresh thyme

Salt

Freshly ground black pepper

NOTES

2 WAYS TO MAKE BROTH

STOVE TOP

1. Combine all ingredients in a large soup pot.
2. Bring to a boil over medium-high heat and then reduce the heat to a simmer, cover, and cook for 4 hours.
3. Strain the broth into another pot or a storage container, and discard the solids. Season with salt.

INSTANT POT

If you have an 8-quart multicooker (such as an Instant Pot), you can really speed up this process. Combine all the ingredients in the pot, cover, and seal. Using the "Manual" function, cook on high for 30 minutes. Leave the broth to sit for 1½ to 2 hours. Strain the broth into another pot or a storage container, and discard the solids. Season with salt.

VEGETABLE BROTH

5 garlic cloves, unpeeled, chopped

5 carrots, unpeeled, chopped

5 celery stalks, chopped

2 bay leaves

1 yellow onion, unpeeled, chopped

1 sweet potato, unpeeled, chopped

½ leek, cut into thirds

½ bunch fresh flat-leaf parsley, chopped

small handful fresh rosemary

14 cups water

1 teaspoon salt

Soup Bowls

You can use more or less broth depending on how big your soup bowl is, but I typically use 1 to 2 cups of broth for a single serving. You can slice or chop the protein and veggies however you like and cook as desired before using in these soup bowls.

Prepare all ingredients as desired, being sure to cook meats thoroughly. Place broth in the bottom of your bowl, and then fill the bowl with any or all of the other ingredients listed.

CHICKEN SOUP BOWL

Chicken bone broth

Chicken

Ginger

Lemon juice

Vegetables

BEEF SOUP BOWL

Beef bone broth

Beef

Scallions

Cilantro

Lime juice

Vegetables

SEAFOOD OR FISH SOUP BOWL

Chicken or vegetable broth

Seafood or fish of choice (salmon, shrimp, scallops, etc.)

Lemon juice

Leeks

Tomatoes

Scallions

NOTES

MEAT, POULTRY, AND FISH

All dishes and bowls are meant to serve 3 to 4 people or meal prep 4 meals. Gauging how much you want to eat of something will also help you know if you need to add or subtract any ingredients. These are fun ideas and bases for you to be creative with when you are healing your gut. Anything can be altered to your liking once you get into your groove. Many of the ingredients can go from one bowl to the next. It is important for this to be easy and taste good at the same time.

Combine all sauce and/or topping ingredients. Pour over protein and cook in a pan or bake in the oven. Feel free to use your oil of choice when searing, roasting, or oven baking.

NOTES

APRICOT CHICKEN

1½ pounds chicken

½ cup fresh apricots

¼ cup cilantro

½ cup green olives

¼ cup honey

TOMATO BASIL CHICKEN

1 to 1½ pounds chicken

1 (15-ounce) can tomatoes

¼ cup fresh basil

½ cup coconut milk

2 cloves garlic

HONEY-BALSAMIC CHICKEN

2 chicken tenderloins

1 tablespoon honey

2 tablespoons balsamic vinegar

COCONUT-HONEY CHICKEN

2 boneless skinless chicken breasts

1 tablespoon coconut oil

½ teaspoon honey

Pinch of ground cinnamon

TURKEY LEGS WITH BRUSSELS SPROUTS AND RAISINS

2 turkey legs

½ cup Brussels sprouts

2 tablespoons olive oil

Fresh herb(s) of choice

¼ cup raisins

PINEAPPLE SALMON

3 salmon fillets

1 cup pineapple

¼ cup fresh mint

Juice of 1 lemon

2 cloves garlic

WILD ALASKAN POLLOCK

2 fillets wild Alaskan pollock or other white fish

2 tablespoons lemon juice

Sea salt, as desired

2 sprigs fresh dill

2 sprigs fresh thyme

WILD SALMON

2 fillets wild salmon or other wild-caught fish

2 tablespoons lemon juice

1 tablespoon cilantro

1 tablespoon parsley

NOTES

BURGER-INSPIRED BOWLS AND DISHES

Any Creation in sandwich form can be converted to your bowl of choice. When you're ready, add a more substantial base such as quinoa , rice, etc. to achieve a similar taste and heartiness to a bun or bread.

Combine all ingredients in a bowl. Form into patties. Grill the patties to your desired doneness, or place them in a pan with about 1 tablespoon oil of choice on the stove.

NOTES

TURKEY PATTIES

1 pound ground turkey

1 egg

1 zucchini, peeled and seeded

½ tablespoon chopped fresh rosemary

½ tablespoon chopped fresh thyme

½ teaspoon sea salt

BREAKFAST BURGERS

1 pound ground beef, bison, or turkey

½ cup finely chopped spinach

⅛ teaspoon sea salt

2 tablespoons herbs/spices of choice

SLIGHTLY SWEET BURGER

1 pound ground beef

½ teaspoon ground cinnamon

1 tablespoon chopped fresh sage

1 tablespoon chopped fresh tarragon

HERBED BURGER

1 pound ground beef

1 tablespoon chopped fresh rosemary

1 tablespoon chopped fresh sage

SIDES AND SNACKS

Sometimes you'll want a little something extra but not necessarily a dessert. Sides and snacks are an easy way to have something on hand at all times. Make note that almost all the Creations in this book can technically fit in the "sides and snack" category, depending on what and how much you're in the mood for.

COCOA ROASTED NUTS

1 (16-ounce) bag nuts

¼ cup honey or maple syrup

2 tablespoons unsweetened cocoa powder

2 tablespoons oil

Coat nuts in honey or syrup and then toss with cocoa powder. Bake at 350°F for 10 to 15 minutes.

GARLIC ALMONDS

2 tablespoons coconut aminos

1 tablespoon garlic powder

1 teaspoon paprika

½ teaspoon pepper

2 cups almonds

Combine all ingredients except the almonds, and then toss with almonds to coat. Bake at 325°F for 20 minutes, shaking them halfway through. Goes well on any Asian-inspired bowl.

FRUIT 'N' CREAM

1 piece fruit of your choice

Almond or coconut milk

Ground cinnamon

Coat fruit in almond or coconut milk, sprinkle with cinnamon, and enjoy.

NOTES

GRAIN-FREE APPLE PIE CEREAL

½ cup dried apples

1 to 2 tablespoons flaxseed

1 to 2 tablespoons walnuts

1 to 2 tablespoons slivered almonds

Sprinkle of ground cinnamon

Sprinkle of sea salt

MARINATED EGGS

10 hard-boiled eggs, peeled

3 tablespoons coconut aminos

3 tablespoons apple cider vinegar

3 cloves garlic

2 tablespoons fresh ginger

Combine all ingredients and add enough water to cover all the eggs. Refrigerate for at least 1 day.

SPAGHETTI SQUASH WITH AVOCADO

1 cooked spaghetti squash

1 avocado

Everything But the Bagel® seasoning

Mash avocado into squash. Sprinkle with seasoning and serve.

CARROT FRIES

Whole carrots, halved lengthwise

Olive oil

Sea salt

Rosemary

Toss carrot slices with a drizzle of olive oil, sea salt, and rosemary. Place on a baking sheet and bake at 400°F for 30 minutes, or until crispy.

DESSERTS

Here are some dessert-inspired dishes to give your palate a little sweet treat. Fruit and compliant nut milks can make even the biggest sweet tooth happy. A little fruit and crunch from a nut can really satisfy anyone.

APPLE COBBLER

½ cup almond flour

⅓ cup coconut flakes

2 tablespoons coconut oil

2 tablespoons maple syrup

1 dash ground cinnamon

3 apples, cut into slices

Mix all ingredients except apples. Spread apples in a baking pan and bake at 350°F for about 20 minutes, or until soft. Sprinkle on topping mixture and bake for an additional 15 minutes at 400°F, until topping is golden.

CHOCOLATE NICE CREAM

2 frozen bananas

2 tablespoons cocoa powder

Combine all ingredients in a small blender. Blend until completely mixed and smooth.

NOTES

WHIPPED CREAM

Whipped cream makes everything taste a little better. It's a simple addition to fruit, as a single-spoon dessert, or even an addition to your favorite beverage. The two whipped cream Creations below will make approximately 4 to 6 servings, depending on how much you use per serving.

In a large bowl, combine all ingredients except 1 tablespoon coconut milk. Use a hand blender to blend until mixture becomes thick and creamy. Add the remaining tablespoon of coconut milk, stir by hand, and enjoy!

NOTE

Once the whipped creams harden, you'll need to soften up with a little more coconut milk due to the addition of the coconut butter. The mixtures can even be placed in the fridge for a few days, but will need to warm to room temperature (and have the liquid coconut milk added) prior to serving. For these reasons, these Creations are best served immediately.

PUMPKIN SPICED WHIPPED CREAM

½ cup + 1 tablespoon full-fat coconut milk

⅓ cup coconut butter, measured and then melted

2 tablespoons pumpkin puree

½ tablespoon coconut sugar

½ teaspoon ground cinnamon

½ teaspoon ground nutmeg

VEGAN WHIPPED CREAM

½ cup + 1 tablespoon full-fat coconut milk, refrigerated overnight

½ teaspoon maple syrup

⅓ cup coconut butter, measured and then melted

NOW WHAT?

So, what comes next?

What comes next is that you continue doing all the work with the foundation you have put into place. I have compiled a ton of references and resources that will be useful to you moving forward. Use them at your own pace and as desired. My goal is to continue serving you in the best ways possible, wherever you are, both online and on your journey. Here is where to find even more *A Gutsy Girl* information and community.

RESOURCE	LINK	NOTES
A Gutsy Girl website	agutsygirl.com	Our main "home"
A Gutsy Girl YouTube channel	www.youtube.com/agutsygirl	New content weekly
Rated-G E-newsletter	https://pages.convertkit.com/7f2076c3f5/1932222263	Exclusive e-newsletter (Rated G for Gutsy)
A Gutsy Girl Instagram	www.instagram.com/agutsygirl/	

A Gutsy Girl podcast	*A Gutsy Girl* podcast wherever you listen to podcasts (Apple Podcasts | Google Podcasts | Spotify | iHeart Radio | RSS)	New episodes released every other week
A Gutsy Girl's Bible private Facebook group	www.facebook.com/groups/agutsygirlbible/	Private Facebook community to connect
TikTok	@agutsygirl	
LinkedIn	www.linkedin.com/in/sarahkayhoffman/	
Pinterest	www.pinterest.com/sarahkayhoffman	Health and healing inspiration via your Pinterest boards
Twitter	https://twitter.com/sarahkayhoffman	

Where to Shop for Food, Supplements, and Lifestyle Items

Preparation is half the battle when it comes to gut health. I shop several times each month (mostly online) and I also regularly shop at multiple local stores for fresh foods and other staples. You may prefer to do one big shopping trip or online grocery order each week. Do whatever you need to do to stock up on the foods that will help you heal.

Below you'll find some of my favorite sources for food, supplements, and lifestyle items.

FOOD

COMPANY	WEBSITE	FOOD ITEMS	SPECIAL SAVINGS
Amazon	amazon.com/shop/agutsygirl	Food, supplement, lifestyle, and more curated by A Gutsy Girl	
Thrive Market (online)	https://bit.ly/agutsygirlbookthrivemarket	Coconut aminos, pasta, pasta sauce, snacks	
Costco (online and physical)	costco.com	Organic meat and poultry, fruits, vegetables, frozen items, peanut butter, almond butter	
Kettle & Fire (online and at grocery stores)	www.kf91trk.com/agutsygirl/	Bone broths	Code AGUTSYGIRL at checkout to save 10%
Daily Harvest	daily-harvest.com	Harvest bowls, smoothies, dairy-free ice cream, lattes, bites	Code AGUTSYGIRL at checkout for special savings

SUPPLEMENTS

COMPANY	WEBSITE	PRODUCT(S)	SPECIAL SAVINGS
Paleovalley	Paleovalley.com	Apple cider vinegar complex, grass-fed beef sticks, Essential C complex, Organ complex	Code AGUTSYGIRL at checkout for 15% off
Perfect Supplements	perfectsupplements.com	Gelatin, D3, Low-FODMAP protein powder, magnesium	Code AGUTSYGIRL for 10% off
Just Thrive Health	justthrivehealth.com	IgG Immune and Digestive Boost, Gluten Away, Immunity Plus, probiotics, prebiotics, K2-7, Gut 4-tify, Just Calm	Code AGUTSYGIRL at checkout for 15% off
Gut Garden	mygutgarden.com	Collagen, digestive enzyme, resistant starch	Code AGUTSYGIRL at checkout for 15% off
FoodMarble	Foodmarble.com	At-home hydrogen + methane breath testing device.	Code GUTSYG at checkout to save 15% off the device +/or FODMAP program
Atrantil	atrantil.com	Bloating and digestive health; many use in conjunction with SIBO	Code GUTSY10 at checkout to save 10%
Amazon	Find in my Amazon store	Dysbiocide	
LMNT	DrinkLMNT.com/AGG	Electrolytes	FREE sampler pack (only pay for shipping)

SUPPLEMENTS (CONTINUED)

COMPANY	WEBSITE	PRODUCT(S)	SPECIAL SAVINGS
Matula Tea	www.matulatea. com/#a_ aid=AGUTSYGIRL	Made specifically for those with *H. Pylori*	

LIFESTYLE

COMPANY	WEBSITE	PRODUCT(S)	SPECIAL SAVINGS
Beautycounter	www.beautycounter. com/sarahhoffman	Makeup, skincare	
Primally Pure	https:// primallypure.com/	Face, body, hair, wellness tools, dry brushes	Code AGUTSYGIRL at checkout for 15% off
Dr. Bronner's	www.drbronner.com/	Pure Castile Liquid Soap	
Wellnesse	wellnesse.com?oid= 1&affid=19	Shampoo, dry shampoo, conditioner, hand sanitizer, toothpaste, dental floss	
Redmond's Earthpaste	redmond.life/ collections/ earthpaste-all	Toothpaste	
AirDoctor Pro	Airdoctorpro.com	Air purifier	Code AGUTSYGIRL at checkout to save up to $300 off your air purifier
AquaTru Water Filter	Aquatruwater.com	Water filter	Code AGUTSYGIRL at checkout to save $150 off your water filter
Branch Basics	links. branchbasics.com	Nontoxic cleaning and laundry	Code AGUTSYGIRL for 15% off Starter Kits

LIFESTYLE (CONTINUED)

COMPANY	WEBSITE	PRODUCT(S)	SPECIAL SAVINGS
doTerra	my.doterra.com/sarahhoffman7	Essential oils, diffusers	
Our Place	fromourplace.com/	The Always Pan	
NOW®	Nowfoods.com	Nuts, seeds, diffuser, essential oils, supplements (their L-Glutamine is one of my favorite brands for pure L-Glutamine)	

Looking for even more recommendations for food, supplements, and lifestyle + savings to accompany? Scan the QR code to be taken to the Bible Resource page.

SACCHARIDES

A saccharide is not some chemical or additive you'll find on a food label. As a matter of fact, *saccharide* is simply another term for carbohydrate. Saccharides are natural, but not everyone understands them, and depending on the type, they can be problematic for the Gutsy Girl. There are four groups of saccharides:

Monosaccharides are the simplest form of sugar. These are carbohydrates that contain a single "ring" and cannot be broken down into any other carbohydrates. They include glucose (dextrose), fructose (levulose), galactose, xylose, and ribose, and they are found in fruits, vegetables, nuts, honey, and some meats.

Disaccharides contain two rings linked together. Common disaccharides include lactose, sucrose, and maltose. Lactose, for example, is a disaccharide made up of one galactose ring and one glucose ring.

Oligosaccharides are a type of carbohydrate that includes three to ten simple sugars linked together. The most common are fructans and galactans.

Polysaccharides are long carbohydrate chains. They are found in starchy carbs like corn, potatoes, rice, bread, pasta, and cereal; in the cellulose in foods like apple and pear skins and spinach; and in oats, beans, nuts, psyllium husks, flaxseed, carrageenan, and carrots and other root vegetables.

In theory, monosaccharides should be the easiest for the Gutsy Girl to digest. Since they are already broken down to their simplest form, our bodies don't need to work as hard to process them. But because we see monosaccharides as the "best option," it can be easy to overindulge. Even "good" things can be harmful if consumed in too large a quantity. For example, fructose is a monosaccharide that should be okay for most Gutsy Girls. But a normal-functioning gut can only process 25 to 50 grams per of fructose at a time, and if you have gut issues that cause fructose malabsorption, your body may only be able to process as little as 1 gram per serving. So while your gut is healing, even monosaccharides like those found naturally in fruit should be portion-controlled and eaten with caution. An apple a day may keep the doctor away—or it may leave your gut feeling miserable!

Lactose is another example of a saccharide that can be harder for those with gut issues to process. Lactose is a disaccharide, with just two compounds. Seems fairly simple, right? So why do so many people have problems digesting lactose?

In order to break the milk sugar lactose down into its two compounds, we need the enzyme lactase to do so. Lactose is not digested until it reaches the small intestine where the hydrolytic enzyme lactase is located. Lactase (β-galactosidase) is a membrane-bound enzyme located in the brush border epithelial cells of the small intestine. Lactase catalyzes the hydrolysis of lactose into its constituent monosaccharides.[1] Therefore, for many people, breaking down lactose is too difficult.

The bottom line is, when the gut is damaged in any way, shape, or form, it is simply not as capable of doing the hard work to break down more complex molecules. If you have IBS or IBD, many foods that are ordinarily deemed "healthy" are composed of structures and enzymes that your body may struggle to break down.jeans

---

[1] https://www.sciencedirect.com/topics/agricultural-and-biological-sciences/disaccharides

And unsurprisingly, more complications bring, well, more complications. Ogliosaccharides, like those found in certain veggies and legumes, no longer have nice, linear-structured rings, and their complexity makes them harder to break down. Before I healed my own gut, I found that nearly every time I would eat Brussels sprouts, cabbage, or broccoli, like clockwork my stomach would instantly feel horrible. I continued to eat them because I thought they were "good for me" (and because I love them!), but I eventually figured out that the raffinose—an ogliosaccharide—found in these types of veggies simply didn't agree with my gut.

Finally, polysaccharides are so complex that they are even more difficult for the digestive system to handle. Digesting polysaccharides involves a variety of enzymes that must first break the polysaccharides into disaccharides, and then into monosaccharides, before the body can begin to use them. As Elaine Gottschall explains, "In a healthy person all these processes work perfectly." But if you have gut-health issues, your body may not produce enough enzymes to digest all the carbohydrates, and undigested carbohydrates will remain in the intestines. "This would normally be no problem," Gottschall notes, "because whatever the body doesn't utilize will end up in the toilet. However, the intestines also have natural inhabitants: Bacteria. The bacteria have been waiting for a long time for such a feast! Lots and lots of disaccharides, their favorite meal! To thank you for the meal, they start to produce large amounts of gas [...] and acids. As a result, the gas pressure in the intestines gets higher and higher. The body wants to relieve itself of the overpressure, and the host (you) starts to burp and fart. Also, the gas is giving the stomach some false signals. The stomach replies by producing more digestive acids. The result for the host: heartburn and throwing up and nausea."[2]

---

[2]*Breaking the Vicious Cycle: Intestinal Health Through Diet*, Elaine Gottschall, MS

HOW TO DIGEST SACCHARIDES

Fortunately, even if you have gut issues, you don't have to give up all saccharides forever. Following a few key pieces of advice can help you safely enjoy saccharides in moderation.

1. When it comes to the foods we are mildly intolerant to, moderation is key. For example, while Brussels sprouts, sweet potatoes, broccoli, and cauliflower used to shred my stomach, if I stick to just ½ cup or less at a time, I'm able to digest them just fine. Proper portion control will allow you to eat the high-quality, beneficial foods that contain saccharides without having to fear getting bloated or having it all run right through you.

2. Enzyme supplements can help give your body the tools it needs to break down saccharides. If I'm craving butternut squash, for example, taking an enzyme (or sometimes even two) beforehand can help me avoid the problems I might have otherwise had.

3. Prepare your food correctly. With certain foods, fermenting them can help improve their digestibility. For example, if a dairy product has been fermented, the amount of lactose in it decreases. This is why fermented yogurt, for example, may be easier for your body to digest than nonfermented milk.

4. Quit with your excuses. Avoiding saccharides is not an excuse to avoid healthy foods like Brussels sprouts and beans while loading up with junk. Processed food, and crap food in general, is filled with saccharides, too, and these don't just disappear from your system overnight. It may take months or even years of committing to a healing diet to make long-term changes in your gut. If you are ready to heal your gut, you'll stop making excuses and do the work— and eventually, many of these saccharides will be your friends again.

WHY IS YOUR GLUTEN-FREE DIET KEEPING YOU MISERABLE?

These days it seems everyone is gluten-free, but for the vast majority, going gluten-free is more of a fad than anything. If you are in the Gutsy club, though, and you're gluten-free, there's probably a very good medical reason for it. There's also a very high possibility that your gluten-free diet is contributing to keeping you miserable.

Why? If you've started your gluten-free journey by reading resources and looking at brand marketing that's geared toward the vast majority of gluten-free people, you're probably doing yourself a major disservice. If you are eating gluten-free for medical reasons, you shouldn't be worrying about calorie counts or any of the other things marketers may be touting on their product packaging. And it's important to realize that the term "gluten-free" on a product doesn't always mean much. If something is labeled "gluten-free," all that means is that it will be free of the protein gluten. But in many instances, gluten-free products are pumped full of alternative ingredients to help them taste and look similar to their gluten-filled counterparts. These alternative ingredients may include things like rice, soy flour, palm oil, sugar, and other things that are definitely *not* helpful for your gut-healing process. When you pick up these boxes at the store, the label clearly demonstrates ingredient complexity. The cookies may be gluten-free, but they're packed full of other ingredients that will likely wreak havoc on your gut.

If you have a gut disorder, you must understand that the gluten-free diet society that is preaching and marketing to you is not the one that is going to heal you forever. If the package says "gluten-free," investigate. And remember that the best gluten-free diet is one that does not come in a package at all.

GLOSSARY

A1C: A blood test that measures blood glucose levels to test for prediabetes or type 2 diabetes.

A Gutsy Girl: It's *you*, my darling!

Autoimmune paleo (AIP): The Paleo Autoimmune Protocol, typically abbreviated AIP, is a powerful strategy that uses diet and lifestyle to regulate the immune system, putting an end to these attacks and giving the body the opportunity to heal.[1]

Bacterial overgrowth of the small intestine: An overgrowth of bacteria that occurs in the small intenstine (SIBO)..

Bowel movement (BM): An act of passing usually solid waste through the rectum and anus.

Bristol Stool Chart: A chart that breaks down stools into seven types and is used to help identify gastrointestinal distress or food sensitivities.

---

[1]https://www.thepaleomom.com/start-here/the-autoimmune-protocol/

Butyrate: A short-chain fatty acid that gut bacteria produces when it breaks down food.

Colonoscopy: A procedure where a long, thin, flexible tool is inserted via the rectum in order to view the bowels and colon.

Complete blood count (CBC): A blood count that includes separate counts for red and white blood cells.

Endoscopy: A procedure where a long, thin, flexible tool called an endoscope is inserted via the mouth to view the esophagus.

Enzymes: Proteins in the body that catalyze biological reactions.

FODMAP: FODMAPs are a classification of carbohydrates (sugars) that don't properly absorb in the gut, in turn they can trigger IBS symptoms."[2]

GAPS Diet: Created by Dr. Natasha Campbell-McBride, the GAPS diet aims to reduce overall inflammation throughout the body by supporting the gut lining through a very specific diet intended to detoxify and restore."[3]

Gastroesophageal reflux disease (GERD): GERD is what acid reflux progresses to, if/when it worsens. It is what occurs when stomach acid reverses back into the esophagus (where it's not supposed to be).[4]

---

[2]https://www.monashfodmap.com/about-fodmap-and-ibs/
[3]https://www.gapsdiet.com/
[4]https://www.mayoclinic.org/diseases-conditions/gerd/

Gastrointestinal (GI): The GI refers to both the upper and lower digestive systems. This is generally considered to start in the mouth (upper) and end in the anus (lower).

Ghrelin: The hormone in your body that indicates hunger.

Hydrochloric acid (HCL): An aqueous solution of hydrogen chloride HCl that is a strong corrosive irritating acid, is normally present in a dilute form in gastric juice, and is widely used in industry and in the laboratory.

Hypothalamic-pituitary-adrenal axis (HPA axis): A neuroendocrine unit that is made up the hypothalamus, pituitary gland, and adrenal glands. This axis plays a key role in the body's response to stress. Though commonly referred to as "adrenal fatigue," the correct term is hypothalamic-pituitary-adrenal axis dysfunction (HPA axis dysfunction, for short).

Inflammatory bowel disease (IBD): either of two inflammatory diseases of the bowel:
    a: CROHN'S DISEASE
    b: ULCERATIVE COLITIS

Intermittent Fasting (IF): Switching between fasting and eating on a regular schedule. There are various methods and cycles used (e.g., 16 hours fasting / 8 hours eating, fasting 12 hours a day / eating 12 hours a day, etc.).

Immunoglobulin E (igE): Antibodies produced in the immune system.

Immunoglobulin G (igG): The most common type of antibody found in blood circulation.

Insoluble fiber: Fiber that cannot be digested by gut bacteria (does not dissolve in water).

Insulin: A hormone released by the pancreas that signals to the body to utilize glucose that has been absorbed from the digestive tract.

symptoms-causes/syc-20361940

Irritable bowel syndrome (IBS): IBS is classified as a syndrome, not a disease. It includes a range of symptoms from constipation to diarrhea, cramping to abdominal pain, and more, but does not cause tissue inflammation (like IBD; inflammatory bowel disease).

L-glutamine: An amino acid known to protect and build the gut lining (the "L" indicates the specific structure of the amino acid used by humans).

Leaky gut syndrome (LGS): Medically correct term includes: Intestinal permeability. It's when the gut lining becomes damaged and what was once a barrier with tight junctions, has now become permeable.

Low-dose naltrexone (LDN): Naltrexone was approved by the FDA in 1984 for the treatment of opioid addiction, used at a standard dose of 50mg to 100mg per day. Low-dose naltrexone comes in doses that are a 10th or less of the standard dose. Most of the research studies have used 4.5mg per day. Doses range from 0.001mg–16mg in clinical practice, and has been used as of recent for conditions such as chronic pain, Crohn's disease, gastritis, ulcerative colitis, SIBO, and more.[5]

Meal spacing (MS): The act of spacing out meals long enough in order to allow a rest and digest cycle.

Microbiome: The community of living bacteria in your digestive tract.

Migrating motor complex (MMC): Occurring approximately every 90 minutes, this is a cycle which takes place in the stomach and small bowl while fasting, and becomes interrupted by eating.[6]

Motility: Intestinal movement.

Mylk: Plant milk like almond, coconut, cashew, and so on. Used as a replacement for dairy milk.

---

[5] https://ldnresearchtrust.org/what-is-low-dose-naltrexone-ldn
[6] https://pubmed.ncbi.nlm.nih.gov/22450306/

NSAIDs: Nonsteroidal anti-inflammatory drugs (ibuprofen, aspirin, naproxen).

Oral Food Challenge (OFC): A medical procedure in which a food is eaten slowly, in gradually increasing amounts, under medical supervision, to accurately diagnose or rule out a true food allergy.[7]

Poo-pourri: Fragrance spray for the toilet.

Prebiotics: Foods that feed gut bacteria.

Probiotics: Foods or supplements that help improve the overall microbiome of the gut by restoring beneficial bacteria that have been depleted.

Processed foods: Foods that have undergone several manipulations from their original state (e.g., potato chips vs. potatoes).

Proline-rich polypeptides (PRPs): First isolated from ovine colostrum (the "first milk" produced by the breasts). Research indicates it helps restore cellular immune functions.

Root-cause analysis (RCA): A method that uses different approaches and techniques to uncover the true (root) cause of any issue.

Short-chain fatty acid (SCFA): Fatty acids that the gut produces such as acetate, propionate, and butyrate. They are important metabolites in maintaining intestinal homeostasis.[8]

Small intestinal bacterial overgrowth (SIBO): When there is excessive bacteria in the small intestine.

Soluble fiber: Fiber that can be digested by bacteria in the large intestine (dissolves in water).

---

[7]https://www.aaaai.org/tools-for-the-public/conditions-library/allergies/what-do-patients-and-caregivers-need-to-know-about
[8]https://pubmed.ncbi.nlm.nih.gov/19939229/#:~:text=A%20proline%2Drich%20polypeptide%20complex,in%20vivo%20and%20in%20vitro.

Specific carbohydrate diet (SCD): A diet that focuses on certain carbohydrates rather than others in order to aid in gut healing. There is an emphasis on fermented yogurt, vegetables, fruits, meats, and nuts.[9]

Spoon Theory: The idea that we are given a finite number of spoons, and each action we complete depletes one of those spoons. Sooner or later, they run out.

Standard American diet (SAD): An acronym developed to define the diet (both macro and micronutrient composition) typical Americans eat. (Note: SAD is also an acronym for seasonal affective disorder, which is depression or low mood related to seasonal changes.)

Synbiotics: A combination of pro- and prebiotics.

Three pillars: The three components *A Gutsy Girl* believes are the foundation of gut healing–diagnosis, diet, and lifestyle.

Ulcerative colitis (UC): A nonspecific inflammatory disease of the colon of unknown cause characterized by diarrhea with discharge of mucus and blood, cramping abdominal pain, and inflammation and edema of the mucous membrane with patches of ulceration.

---

[9]https://www.nimbal.org/education/the-specific-carbohydrate-diet-/definition-and-history

WHAT IS CARRAGEENAN?

Carrageenan is a controversial ingredient used in many packaged foods and beverages.

At its most basic level, carrageenan is a seaweed. So, you may be wondering, what's wrong with seaweed? First, the carrageenan in most packaged foods is a far cry from the seaweed you'll find in the ocean. According to Chris Kresser, "Carrageenan-containing seaweeds have been used for centuries in food preparations for their gelling proper-ties, but the refined, isolated carrageenan found in modern processed foods has raised concerns in the health-conscious online community."[1]

Additionally, carrageenans might not work for you if you have IBS or IBD, because they are a polysaccharide (see page 258).

According to an in-depth Cornucopia Institute report, "Many indi-viduals experiencing gastrointestinal symptoms (ranging from mild 'belly bloat,' to irritable bowel syndrome, to severe inflammatory bowel disease) have noticed that eliminating carrageenan from the diet leads to profound improvements in their gastrointestinal health."[2]

Carrageenan may be found in a wide range of store-bought foods, including ice cream, coffee creamer, candy, coffee drinks, deli meats, cottage cheese, yogurt, cream cheese, sour cream, almond milk, coco-nut milk, dips, juices, and more. As always, I am a huge advocate for reading labels. Read them carefully, and when you don't know what something is, question it!

---

[1] http://chriskresser.com/harmful-or-harmless-carrageenan/
[2] http://www.cornucopia.org/wp-content/uploads/2013/02/Carrageenan-Report1.pdf

INDEX

ABOUT THE AUTHOR

Sarah Kay Hoffman is the founder of *A Gutsy Girl* (agutsygirl.com) which is an online community geared toward women who are looking for reasonable approaches to healing IBS, IBD, SIBO, and all things gut-focused. What began as an online journal documenting the day-to-day with one health issue after the next, would become less story-focused and more research- and journalism-based. Today, Sarah seeks out highly detailed information and then condenses it in digestible ways for women worldwide.

Sarah graduated from the University of Minnesota with a degree in marketing, English, and mass communications. After years of struggling with her own health issues and understanding there must be more to healing than the answers she was given, she went on to study at the Institute for Integrative Nutrition adding a CHC (Certified Health Coach) certification to her education. She began devoting every spare second to studying and researching (and practicing!) all things gut health and gut healing.

Today she spends 100% of her career-focused time on *A Gutsy Girl*, doing everything from speaking to companies worldwide on gut health and the inspiration for achieving it, to researching, writing, and creating tools like her 90-day gut healing journal, *Healing Blooms from Within*, comprehensive *Beginner's Guide to Gut* Healing e-course, and this book, for women worldwide. She is the author of *The Leaky Gut Meal Plan: 4 Weeks to Detox and Improve Digestive Health* along with several e-books and other guides.

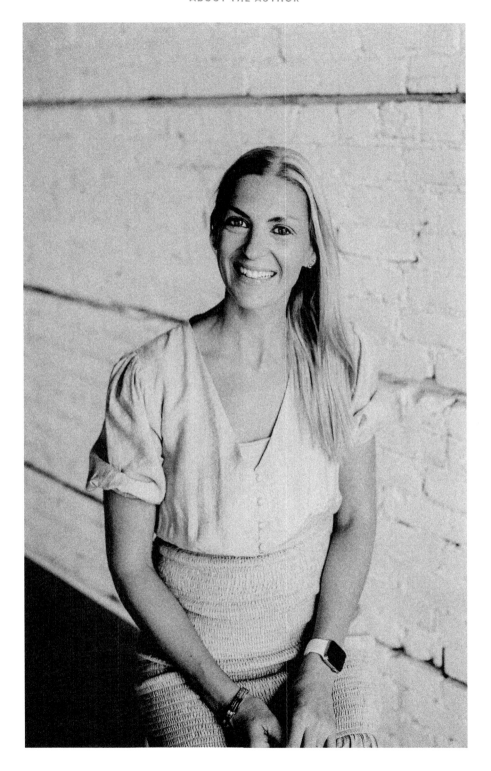

When Sarah is not giving back to the Gutsy community, she is writing on a more personal level at *A Thyme for Milk and Honey* (athymeformilk andhoney.com), working on a new start-up business (thymeonmain.com) with her business partner, traveling, drinking lattes, reading her Bible, enjoying life in a small town, and soaking up all the love that is her husband, three adorable children, peekapoo and two great Danes, family, and friends.

A Gutsy Girl teaches, preaches, and lives by the motto:

Heal your gut. Heal your life.

Email: sarahkay@agutsygirl.com
Instagram: @agutsygirl

Speaking, brand partnerships,
and all other opportunities: opportunities@agutsygirl.com

Printed in Great Britain
by Amazon

79363214R00160